Doing Things

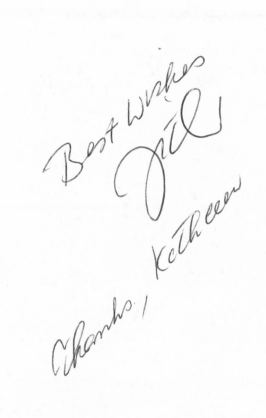

A musician must make music, an artist must paint, a poet must write, if he is to be ultimately at peace with himself. What a man can be he must be.

ABRAHAM MASLOW, Motivation and Personality

Doing Things

*A Guide to Programing Activities
for Persons with Alzheimer's Disease
and Related Disorders*

Jitka M. Zgola

The Johns Hopkins University Press
Baltimore and London

*This book was prepared under the propriety
of the Société Alzheimer Society of Ottawa-Hull.*

© 1987 The Johns Hopkins University Press
Printed in the United States of America on acid-free paper

The Johns Hopkins University Press
2715 North Charles Street
Baltimore, Maryland 21218-4319
The Johns Hopkins Press Ltd., London

Originally published in hardcover and paperback, 1987
04 03 02 01 00 99 98 97 96 95   9 8 7 6 5

Library of Congress Cataloging-in-Publication Data

Zgola, Jitka M.
  Doing things.

  Bibliography: p. 137
  Includes index.
  1. Alzheimer's disease—Patients—Rehabilitation. 2. Alzheimer's
disease—Patients—Recreation. 3. Occupational therapy for the
aged. 4. Day care centers for the aged. I. Title. [DNLM:
1. Alzheimer's Disease—rehabilitation. 2. Day Care. WM 220 Z63d]
RC523.Z46 1987   618.97′683   86-46280
ISBN 0-8018-3466-X (alk. paper)
ISBN 0-8018-3467-8 (pbk.)

A catalog record for this book is available from the British Library.

Contents

Foreword

We each have things to do that fill our day. We dress ourselves and perform our household chores. We care for our children or write our mother. We repair telephones or supervise secretarial pools or design electrical parts for computers. We have hobbies—bowling or partying, model making or stamp collecting. These things occupy major portions of our days and without them we would soon become so restless and bored that we would search for new friends or tasks or hobbies. These things help to define who we are. We say of ourselves, "I am a surgeon," "I am a student," or "I am a homemaker."

The cruel course of a dementing illness takes away our ability to do familiar things. We give up our job only to find that we can no longer enjoy our hobbies either. We cannot get our clothes arranged right side out and someone must dress us. We get lost in the garden, digging up the flowers and leaving the weeds. We forget the grandchildren's names or whether our spouse is still alive. Fear and anxiety make a gentle wife into a shrew. Damage to the brain makes a husband deny that the house he built is his home. Some people fight these losses—stubbornly driving long after it becomes dangerous or "doing their job" when they are only shuffling torn bits of paper. Others retreat into apathy, seeing the world with empty eyes.

Professionals caring for people with dementing illness theorize that the loss of tasks and roles takes away identity. And for individuals who have lost almost all the ability to plan, initiate, or carry out activities, much of the day becomes empty, vacant time. Pacing, fiddling, and repetitious questions may be an effort to fill the void. These people must be helped to find activities that restore a sense of self and a sense of worth.

But what things can these individuals do? Clearly, they can't do what they used to do. Simplified tasks often turn out to be childish, communicating that one's new role is "helpless invalid" or "stupid child." Other tasks turn out to be too difficult and precipitate agitated or angry outbursts. Families and professionals ask, "What to do all day?"

The most successful congregate programs, both adult day care and residential care, have found activities that replace the tasks that have been lost, that support positive roles and make successes possible. Participants in these programs consistently make friends with other participants, seem more confident, happy, and relaxed, and behave in more socially appropriate ways. Although the devastations of the underlying disease have not changed, it is clear that doing things—therapeutic things—significantly improves the quality of life for those with dementing illnesses.

Doing Things answers our questions, "What can we do to enable those in our care to keep on doing things?" "How do we enable them?" "Why do some things work and others not?" It is written for programs in congregate settings, but its insights translate easily into care for the person living at home. It is not a list of ideas for activities; it provides an understanding of the working of the impaired mind and of effective approaches.

We now know that life can be bearable, and sometimes filled with laughter, love, and joy despite the devastations of dementing illnesses. *Doing Things* is a major contribution to our knowledge of this kind of care.

Nancy L. Mace, Coauthor, *The 36-Hour Day*

Preface and Acknowledgments

This book describes the experiences of the staff and clients of "Day Away," the day-program component of the Alzheimer "Day Away" and Home Assistance programs. It is sponsored by the Société Alzheimer Society of Ottawa-Hull and is funded jointly by this society and the Ontario ministries of Health and Community and Social Services.

It is not within the scope of this book to discuss the administration, referral, and admission procedures pertaining to "Day Away." The primary focus of this book is management of and activities for cognitively impaired persons. Those readers who would like more information about the administrative structure of the program will be interested in the descriptive evaluation of "Day Away." This evaluation was completed in January 1986. Copies of the evaluation are available from the Ontario Government Book Store, 880 Bay Street, Toronto, Ontario, Canada M7A 1N8.

Alzheimer's disease affects both men and women. In this book, therefore, masculine and feminine pronouns are used in alternate chapters.

My thanks go to Fran Hadley, R.N., coordinator of the Alzheimer "Day Away" and Home Assistance programs, whose drive and initiative turned an idea into a reality, and to the staff—Allyn Heyes, R.N., assistant coordinator; Gill Michelin, social worker; Doreen Haydon, family support worker; Pat Silverman, voluntary coordinator of volunteers; and Dan Déry and Roy Snider, of Home Assistance—who have all, through their work in the programs, contributed to the ideas expressed here.

The program would not run without a corps of dedicated volunteers. My thanks go to them all, not only for supporting the operation of the program but also for bringing in their own insights, which have helped to keep the program fresh and dynamic. Appreciation must also be expressed to the clients of "Day Away" and their families, whose experiences are described in the following pages.

Thanks for their encouragement, their technical input, and their editorial advice are due to Anne Opzoomer, O.T. (C), M.Sc., registrar of the Ontario College of Occupational Therapists; to Guy Proulx, Ph.D., C.Psych., formerly head of neuropsychology at Élisabeth Bruyère Health Center, Ottawa, now director of Psychological Services at the Baycrest Center, Toronto; and to W. B. Dalziel, M.D., F.R.C.P. (C), associate professor of medicine, head of the Division of Geriatrics, University of Ottawa, and head of the Geriatric Assessment Program, Ottawa Civic Hospital. A special thank you is extended to Bonnie Evans, who tidied up the text of the final draft.

Madeleine Honeyman, founder and president of the Société Alzheimer Society of Ottawa-Hull, must be recognized for her major contribution to the birth of both the "Day Away" program and the Home Assistance program.

The preparation of this book was supported, in part, by a publications grant from the Canadian Occupational Therapy Foundation. This foundation's support is gratefully acknowledged.

A very sincere thank you goes to my family, who gave moral support to this project. Bernie read numerous "final" drafts and maintained an overall good humor. Natalie and Adam learned to take over many new responsibilities and fend for themselves in many ways.

Doing Things

Introduction

*A Program Specifically for
Persons with Alzheimer's Disease*

Day programs provide elderly and disabled persons with an opportunity to be active, to experience success and achievement, and to interact meaningfully with others. Unfortunately, access to these valuable services is often limited for persons with Alzheimer's disease (AD).[1] Many conventional day care centers are reluctant to admit them on the grounds that conventional facilities are not equipped or staffed to deal with some of the behaviors characteristically attributed to clients who have a diagnosis of AD. The most common of these are the tendency to wander, unpredictable and sometimes disruptive behavior, and the inability to follow through with tasks independently. For the AD client, a setting that does not accommodate his or her disabilities can be anxiety provoking and distressing. Forced to stay at home, he or she may be relegated to inactivity and social isolation, while the caregiver is denied the respite that he or she so badly needs.

The Alzheimer's "Day Away" program in Ottawa, Canada, was established to fill this gap. Housed in a local community health center, it offers one day per week of therapeutic activity and social interaction to a total of thirty-two clients (eight per day) with moderate to severe dementia. The aims of the program are to maintain the highest possible level of function among persons with AD and to provide a full day of respite to their caregivers.[2] The program is designed on the basis of current knowledge regarding the neurobehavioral manifestations of the disease and their effects on the individual's ability to function. The physical, social, and operational environment accommodates the clients' disabilities and helps the clients capitalize on their strengths. With this approach, much of the clients' anxiety and fear of failure or embarrassment is removed, and many of the disruptive and perplexing behaviors associated with AD are either eliminated or controlled.

Doing Things is an outgrowth of this innovative program. The title reflects one of the major tenets in "Day Away"'s developing philosophy: we all have an inherent need to do things. We do things to define ourselves as individuals, to exert control over our environment, and to develop and secure meaningful relationships with others. Alzheimer's disease gradually erodes a person's ability to engage in many of the activities that fulfill these basic psychosocial needs. It then becomes the responsibility of the program staff to offer the client alternatives that enable him or her to continue with meaningful activity.

This manual describes the overall approach to programing used at "Day Away." It is intended to serve as a guide to workers and volunteers who plan and carry out activity programs within the community for persons with AD or other dementing conditions. Although the administrative structure of other programs may vary depending on available facilities and existing programs, the information and techniques outlined here should help workers address the special needs of their clients. This information is also applicable to the home setting. Program staff help families and caregivers identify those things that the client can do. At a time when the client's deteriorating skills are most obvious, this positive attitude can be very important.[3] Program directors in nursing homes and homes for the aged may also find this information helpful when planning for their demented residents.

The book begins with an overview of the neurobehavioral aspects of the disease. It describes the characteristic perceptual, cognitive, and motor deficits that affect the person with AD and outlines how these deficits may interfere with his or her ability to function. It also identifies the skills that clients most often retain. Because so much of the activity in the program relates to the stewardship of the clients' psychosocial needs, these needs are reviewed in a separate chapter. The book suggests techniques for arranging the environment and choosing and presenting activities. A selection of demonstrative activities used at "Day Away" is described in detail. The book also outlines some of the techniques used to manage difficult behavior and reduce anxiety among clients in the program.

1 The Neurobehavioral Aspects of Alzheimer's Disease

*Why Doesn't She Want to Do Anything?
or Why Does She Get into Such a Mess
When She Tries to Do Something?*

An effective program must be geared to the particular strengths and weaknesses of its clients. Insight into the process affecting the person with Alzheimer's disease is particularly important because the disabilities are not always apparent on first encounter, and the client's anomalous behavior may be perplexing to the uninformed observer.

Despite having a normal appearance, the client may have difficulty performing many commonplace tasks. She may respond inappropriately to questions or may have difficulty finding her way around a familiar building or neighborhood. She may be reluctant or even become hostile when asked to do certain things. On the other hand, she may perform some tasks flawlessly. These inconsistencies in behavior can be very disconcerting to those caring for her and are often frustrating to the client. One gentleman at "Day Away" has explained the feeling as one of having been betrayed by his brain, which "somehow short-circuited on him."

The condition is, in fact, a physical disorder. The disease produces changes in the cerebral cortex, which is the outer layer of the brain and the part most highly developed in humans.[1] These changes are characterized by deficits in the

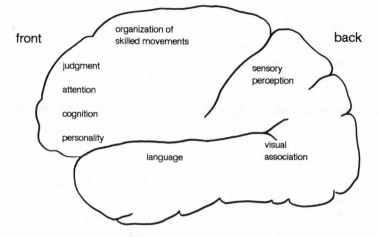

front

back

organization of
skilled movements

judgment

attention

cognition

personality

sensory
perception

visual
association

language

A simplified representation of the distribution of cortical functions
on the cerebral cortex.

affected individual's memory, language, perception,
organization of movement, ability to abstract, attention,
and judgment.[2] Just as the person with a muscular disease
has difficulty moving her limbs, the person with AD has difficulty performing these intellectual functions.

Even a simple situation, such as being asked to make a
bed, requires the use of many of these functions.

- One must understand the verbal command and
  remember what one has been asked to do.
- One must conceptualize the task in abstract terms, not
  taking the word *make* literally.
- One must organize the task in a logical sequence, i.e.,
  strip the bed, smooth the bottom sheet, fluff up and place
  the pillows, etc., ending with a final smoothing of the
  bedspread.
- If the task is to be completed successfully, one must keep
  to the logical sequence of the task, going from one stage
  to the next in the most efficient manner while keeping
  track of the objective and filtering out unimportant
  stimuli.

- Throughout the task, one relies on one's ability to perceive accurately the things one sees and touches.
- Judgment comes into play as one encounters problems, makes decisions about alternatives, and foresees the consequences of each alternative. For example, a sheet caught on a tack in the box spring will rip if pulled out and must be unhooked carefully.
- When the job is finished, one evaluates the quality of the work realistically.

For the individual with impaired memory, judgment, perception, and planning skills, even such a simple task can become a major undertaking. Her fear of failure can be immobilizing. The effort she makes to check and double-check her work can leave her tired and vulnerable to frustration and may even lead to catastrophic reactions on her part.

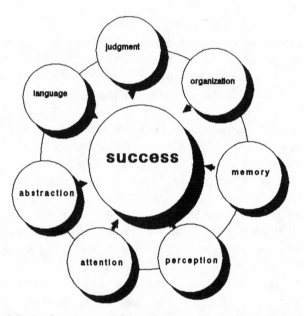

Success in performing many complex tasks depends upon the interplay of all the cognitive functions shown. If any of these functions is impaired, successful completion of the task is jeopardized.

It is impossible to make generalizations, since the disease affects individuals differently depending on which parts of the cortex are most affected and on the extent of the disease, but the most common deficits can be described.

Memory

Memory problems are usually among the first to be noticed. Initially the person, aware of her failing memory, uses aids such as notes to remind herself.[3] Eventually, though, even this ability is lost. Personal items are misplaced or hidden and forgotten. "The pot boiled dry on the stove" is a classic example in Alzheimer literature. So is the failure to recall the names of friends and even family members. Not all aspects of memory are affected equally, however. At times the person may remember things with amazing accuracy. Memory is a complex process and involves a combination of four parameters: functions, modalities, processes, and types of material.[4]

Functions can be divided into three categories: immediate recall, recent memory, and remote memory.[5] Immediate recall refers to the recollection of events immediately following their occurrence. Recent memory refers to the recollection of events occurring within a matter of minutes. Remote memory refers to the recollection of events in the distant past, months to years. These three functions of memory are affected differentially. Immediate recall and recent memory seem to be the most vulnerable; remote memory seems to be the least affected. Loss of recent memory results in the continual repetition of questions which caregivers find so taxing and which severely limits the client's ability to learn new material or acquire new skills.

Modalities are the sensory systems whereby the material remembered was experienced. These are: visual, auditory, and tactile.[6] Most people realize that they tend to remember material experienced through one sense better than they do material experienced via another. For example, one person may have a better memory for things she has read, while another may find it easier to remember things she has heard. Most people, including clients with AD, perform best when material to be remembered is presented to a variety of modalities. One such multisensory experience is walking through a market and reinforcing the memory of things seen by talking about each one as it is observed.

Observation of clients with AD suggests an additional modality that relates to emotional experience: emotionally charged experiences are generally retained but may be recalled in a somewhat distorted fashion.[7] It happens quite frequently that a new client who has been anxious throughout the day retains a negative impression of the program. She may account for her negative feelings by telling her husband that no one paid attention to her or that she did nothing all day.

Four processes that may be identified with memory are: registration, storage, retrieval, and retention.[8] Memory disorders may be related to dysfunction in any of these processes. The client may be unable to respond to a memory item because the material did not register. This is basically a problem of attention. Her brain may be unable to store the information that did register. She may be unable to call upon the item that has been stored. Or, she may be able to retain the stored information for only a finite period of time before it is lost.

Observation of clients in the program suggests that retrieval problems are especially frustrating because they make the clients acutely aware of their inability to remember. Visual and verbal cues are very useful under these circumstances. This is probably why "finish the proverb" games are so popular. The first few words of the saying will trigger the memory, and the client experiences the satisfaction of remembering.

Finally, memory may be mediated by the type of material involved. This material can be either verbal or nonverbal.[9] Material that is only verbal is often difficult for clients to retain. Material containing both verbal and nonverbal elements seems to be retained better. Therefore, verbal material should be reinforced by action and by visual clues, and vice versa.

When evaluating a client's memory, it is important for us to remember that our casual appraisal can be confounded by a variety of factors. The client may be experiencing per-

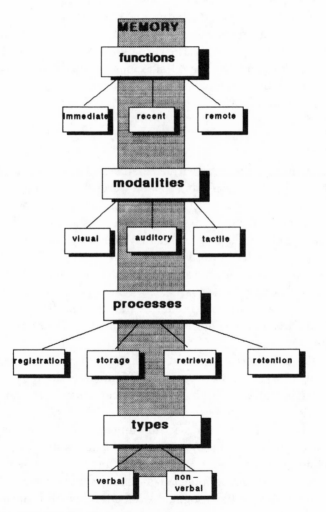

Parameters that mediate memory.

ceptual and language problems that can make her appear as though she does not remember things accurately.

Common forgetfulness can be a nuisance or an embarrassment. Memory loss, however, is devastating. Imagine the anxiety the client must feel upon entering a room and not recognizing the people who greet her, not knowing how she got there, how she is going to get home, or whether her loved ones know where she is. Another consequence of memory loss is that it robs the individual of her past.

The client's memory deficit can put a tremendous strain on the caregiver, as well. The caregiver may reassure and inform the client, but the relief is short-lived. As the client forgets, anxiety wells up again, and the same reassurances and information must be repeated over and over.

Language

The majority of persons with Alzheimer's disease experience little difficulty articulating spoken words, but language problems unrelated to sensory, motor, or intellectual deficits are common. These are referred to as aphasia. The earliest evidence of language problems in Alzheimer's disease is usually difficulty in word-finding.[10] This inability to recall the appropriate word is called anomia. The individual will often "talk around" the issue, trying to identify the object by its use or location. In the latter stages of the disease, this circumlocution can deteriorate into a jumble of rambling non sequiturs.

Paraphasia is another type of language disturbance commonly observed in victims of AD. Clients interchange words that sound alike or fall into the same category.[11] For example, *nurse* for *purse,* or *mother* for *wife.* If the person's speech is well articulated, with good flow and appropriate intonation, the presence of a significant language disturbance may not be apparent at first. Paraphasias can make the client appear to be quite deranged or, at least, very confused. Active, informed listening, however, often reveals that the client does, in fact, know what she is trying to say, and that

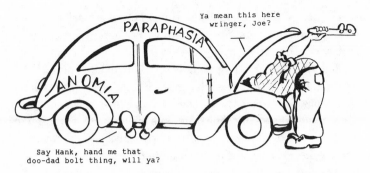

Everyone has, at one time or another, experienced episodes of anomia and paraphasia.

she is just coming out with the wrong words. The challenge to the listener lies in figuring it out!

The inability to express oneself, to share feelings, needs, observations, and ideas, can cause a person to withdraw and give up or become angry and frustrated. Communication difficulties create a serious rift between the person with AD and those around her.

Perception

Perception is the ability to interpret, meaningfully, sensory information coming into the brain via the sensory organs. Perceptual problems in AD are manifest in a variety of ways. The most common ones are visuospatial difficulties, which involve the inability to perceive direction, distance, and the spatial relationship of objects to one's body and to each other;[12] and agnosia, which is the inability to recognize familiar objects and symbols.[13] Disturbances in body awareness, the conceptual image of one's body and its organization, may also be observed.

Visuospatial problems cause the person to become lost, even in familiar surroundings. She may be unable to distinguish between markings on a flat surface and three-dimensional objects or to judge distance. As a result, she may step carefully over lines on the floor or bump into furniture. Such problems can make the person feel very uncomfortable and anxious. The discomfort is often expressed as resistance, hostility, or aggression.

The true nature of agnosia is still the focus of much lively debate. Whether each sense affected is the manifestation of a separate entity or whether, as a group, the agnosias are a combination of other problems of cognition remains to be determined. For the purposes of this discussion, however, I will adhere to the definition outlined above.

Agnosia can affect any of the senses. A person with visual agnosia may have difficulty identifying a comb visually but, permitted to handle it, will recognize it as a useful object and will be able to use it appropriately. A person with tactile agnosia finds it difficult to interpret touch without visual clues. This is particularly significant, as an unexpected touch outside the client's field of vision may be very uncomfortable or even threatening.

Alexia, the inability to understand written language, is sometimes associated with agnosia. Many people with AD can read aloud fluently but have no understanding of the material they are reading.

As a result of disturbed body awareness, the person becomes unable to conceptualize how her body parts are organized in relation to one another. This makes grooming and dressing very difficult. In the latter stages of the disease, the client may not even be able to identify parts of her body while looking at them. The ability to interpret accurately sensory messages coming from within the body, such as localizing pain or interpreting the message from a full bladder, may be lost.

The Organization of Movement

Skilled movement demands the ability to translate ideas into motor actions, to organize actions and events in a logical sequence, and to combine parts of objects to form a whole. Persons with AD may experience difficulty in all these areas. They may not be able to imitate a simple posture or respond accurately to a verbal command such as "Cross your fingers." They may put their clothes on in the wrong order or be unable to solve a simple puzzle. These clients tend to depend on "overlearned" patterns of movement which do not require conscious thought or sequencing.[14] As a result, new activities or sequences of tasks can be disconcerting.

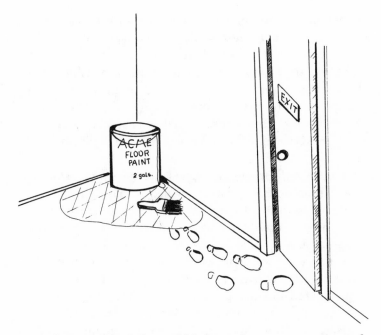

Even the most straightforward job demands some sequencing and planning skills.

Abstract Thought

With Alzheimer's disease, insight and the ability to form and understand abstract concepts diminish.[15] The person may take literally the common metaphors or figures of speech used in ordinary conversation. This can lead to frustrating misunderstandings. Because she is unable to appreciate the implications of a situation such as a lost credit card, she may appear to be apathetic in her lack of concern. The person may deny the existence of disease. Denial of this type cannot be resolved through reasoning. It tends to be absolute and may lead to very unpleasant confrontations when medical help or special programs are offered.

Attention

Attention is a very complex phenomenon whose domain ranges from simple vigilance through concentration and higher levels of selective attention. It is said to be a major frontier of the neurosciences. There remains much to be defined and redefined in this area. For the purposes of this discussion, I will define attention as the individual's ability to initiate, maintain, and terminate an activity appropriately. In AD we may see disturbances in all of these functions.

Inertia is the inability to get started on things. This is often wrongly perceived as indolence or apathy, but the truth is that the person does not have a "starter button." Something external must be brought to bear in order to get her started. A visual or tactile cue will often help.

Once the person is involved in an activity, she may have difficulty staying with the task. She may be drawn to a salient detail and disregard the rest of the situation: for instance, she may persistently pick at a breadcrumb instead of clearing off the whole table. She may be unable to focus her attention on any one thing. Her attention span may be very short, and she may lose interest before the task is completed.

Perseveration refers to the client's inability to stop once she has started a pattern of behavior. The individual may persist in the established pattern—she may wash the dishes over and over—until an external event brings her to a halt. Perseveration may also result in the individual's inability to control the force and persistence of her actions: she may rub right through a sheet of paper when trying to erase a mark. Her playful tap may escalate into a barrage of painful slaps.

Judgment

Impaired judgment may result in a person showing little regard for social conventions. She may not recognize sound advice when it is offered or be able to decide on an effective course of action when faced with an unfamiliar or emergency situation. This leaves her vulnerable to any number of dangers, both at home and in the community. It also makes her prone to the social faux pas that can be embarrassing for everyone concerned.

These descriptions should be used only as a means of understanding observed behavior. Accurate, ongoing evaluation is essential to determine actual strengths and deficits. Adhering to stereotypes about clients with Alzheimer's disease can create preconceptions about the clients' limitations, foster learned helplessness on the clients' part, and squelch whatever initiative and compensatory mechanisms the clients retain. Disability may be anticipated but not presumed until it has been observed and the clients' inability to overcome it independently has been demonstrated.

2　Evaluation

*Finding out What He Can Do and
What He Can't Do, Why, and What
He Does as an Alternative*

Chapter 1 reviewed the difficulties most commonly experienced by persons with Alzheimer's disease. The plan for an individual client, however, must be based on an accurate evaluation of his condition and his strengths, deficits, and needs. This information is obtained from a number of sources, including neurological and physical examination, neuropsychological testing, psychiatric review, functional evaluation, and social history. Evaluation of the client's home environment helps staff transfer the benefits obtained at the day program into the client's home.

Medical Examination

Neurological examination contributes to the diagnostic process by ruling out the presence of central nervous disorders that may be arrestable or treatable. Physical examination can confirm that dementia exists or discover reversible conditions that mimic the presentation of dementia.[1] The most common of these are hypothyroidism, malnutrition, and side effects from medication. These and a variety of other conditions can be screened out by a comprehensive medical assessment and laboratory tests.

Less than 10 percent of all dementias are completely reversible with medical treatment. However, it is important to realize that illness can indirectly affect mental function and result in an overall decline in the patient's functional cognitive abilities. Although the dementia may not have been cured, treatment of the reversible elements may bring about an overall improvement in the patient's ability to function. As persons with AD have no "brain reserve," they are particularly susceptible to superimposed acute confusional states resulting from other illnesses. It is, therefore, important that these illnesses be investigated and treated. A sudden deterioration in cognitive function must be brought to the attention of a physician and not simply be attributed to an irreversible progressive dementia.[2]

Neuropsychological Testing

Neuropsychological testing isolates specific perceptual and cognitive domains and evaluates each one objectively in relation to standardized norms. It aids in the formulation of a diagnosis by identifying constellations of cognitive symptoms that are characteristic of Alzheimer's disease.[3] Particularly useful to the program planner, however, is the way in which neuropsychology defines observed behavior in terms of specific neurological dysfunction. Information such as "The client cannot perform this function because this particular part of his cortex has been damaged" helps us account for the client's difficulties and develop a rational program strategy. It can also give us a clearer picture of the strengths that the client may be encouraged to exploit.[4]

Psychiatric Review

Psychiatric review is especially important when any emotional problem is suspected. The psychiatrist has an important role in confirming the presence of dementia, since depression, especially in the elderly, may present itself as dementia by seriously affecting a person's cognitive function.[5] Depression may also be associated with the dementing process and further impair the client's cognitive and functional abilities. If the depression, which is usually treatable, is alleviated, an improvement in function is usually observed.[6]

Functional Evaluation

Functional evaluation is intended to provide an accurate picture, not only of what the client is capable of doing but also of what he does, in fact, do and how he does it. Many clients call upon a variety of resources in order to achieve at a level higher than would be anticipated on the basis of standardized neuropsychological testing.[7] Each person's personality will determine how he copes with disability. Functional evaluation outlines the client's level of achievement in terms of basic senses and functions, mobility, self-care, independent living, behavior and interpersonal relations, and cognitive function.

Assessment of basic senses and functions takes note of physical handicaps or deficits in basic senses, muscle strength, joint range of motion, and equilibrium. Information from the medical examination is correlated with observations of the client's abilities to determine if and how existing deficits actually interfere with his ability to function.

Mobility includes the client's ability to ambulate, transfer, use assistive devices (such as wheelchairs, canes, or walkers), and negotiate obstacles, stairs, and rough ground. Evaluation of mobility should include observations of the physical and perceptual impediments that the client encounters while moving about. It should also document the circumstances under which he is best able to achieve.

Self-care refers to dressing, feeding, personal hygiene and grooming, toileting, and sleeping. Note should be taken of schedules and patterns of incidents where toileting or sleeping difficulties occur. Again, it is important to document the type of impediments that the client encounters and the circumstances under which he is able to achieve maximum independence.

Independent living refers to the use of transportation, money management, shopping, housekeeping, meal preparation, and the use of community and social resources. Observations should reflect the actual demands made on the client in his current life situation and his ability to respond to them.

Behavior and interpersonal relations relate to the client's ability to communicate, his predominant affect and emotional status, and the quantity and quality of his social contacts and family ties. The evaluation in this area also describes the client's response to frustration and conflict, as well as the soundness of his judgment and insight.

Evaluation of cognitive function includes basic perceptual-motor abilities, memory, and orientation. Information from neuropsychological tests and other standardized tests, such as the Hierarchic Dementia Scale (H.D.S.),[8] is related to observations. It is important to note any compensatory mechanisms the client uses to overcome cognitive or perceptual deficits.

What can the client do?

What does the client do?

How does he/she do it?

Which parts of the task is the client unable to do?

Why is he/she unable to do them?

Where does he/she perform best?

When does he/she perform best?

The seven Ws of functional evaluation.

Social History

A social history gives insight into social status, aspirations, and standards against which the client judges himself and is judged by his peers. It also provides a picture of the client's previous personality and identifies the changes that have occurred as a result of his illness.

Environment

A separate evaluation of the client's environment and his interaction with it is also important. A description of living arrangements will help identify supports, demands, and potential sources of stress.

Program planners can use all of the foregoing information to tailor programs to the needs of individual clients. At "Day Away," this information is collected in an evaluation protocol specifically designed for the program (appendix C) and is supplemented with the Hierarchic Dementia Scale and the Family Burden Index.[9]

Ongoing Evaluation

Initial evaluation must be complemented by ongoing, informed observation. This ongoing evaluation should be documented in notes made by program staff which describe the activities of each client in this program. Without this type of record it would be difficult to track, objectively, changes in the client's functional abilities. These notes may be supplemented by a journal in the form of a small notebook that travels between home and the program with each client. The program staff and the client's family can use this journal as a means of communicating significant events and information on a regular basis.

3   Programing to the Clients' Strengths

Despite the potential deficits described in chapter 1, some very important abilities and strengths are characteristically retained by persons with Alzheimer's disease. Program planners must pay special attention to these strengths, because they form the basis of the clients' functional abilities. In addition, some characteristics of persons with AD can be used to advantage in planned activities. Programs should take maximal advantage of the ability to perform overlearned or habitual tasks, primary motor and sensory functions, emotional awareness, remote memory, and the tendency to perseverate.

Habitual Skills

Once a sequence of actions has been learned and practiced, it becomes habitual and no longer requires planning, organization, and modulation. The sequence becomes an "automatic program," which the person calls up in response to a specific environmental stimulus. Many clients depend almost exclusively on these habitual skills to perform the activities of daily living.

Even habitual skills may eventually become lost to the

person with AD, but the loss tends to be patchy, and some very remarkable abilities may remain intact. A client may be able to play the piano long after she has lost more simple skills.

Clients' habitual skills can be used to advantage in an activity program. For example, given a tea towel in one hand and a cup in the other and directed to a rack of washed dishes, even a very handicapped client may be able to dry dishes without further instructions.

Social skills are another form of "automatic programing." Many clients can function comfortably in structured social situations, such as introductions, teas, and meals,

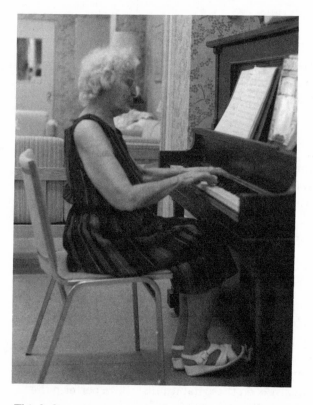

This lady continues to enjoy her skill at the piano and the pleasure it brings to others.

because they are confident in their ability to call up the appropriate responses.[1]

At times, habitual patterns get in the way. An environmental cue may trigger a familiar but inappropriate sequence of behavior in the client which may be embarrassing or even hazardous. Habitual skills tend to be rigid and tolerate no interruption or deviation. If a client is distracted from a task, she may not be able to return to it easily or may have to start again from the beginning.

Primary Motor Function

Although the ability to conceptualize, organize, initiate, and modulate movement may become impaired, primary motor functions such as strength, dexterity, and muscular control are usually retained. Clients can perform a variety of fairly demanding tasks if each step is pointed out, instructions are given precisely, and compensation is made for perceptual problems.

Primary Sensory Function

Primary sensory function is also generally unimpaired. Although the individual may not always make sense of all that she sees, hears, touches, smells, and tastes, she can still derive pleasure from pleasant sensations or be repulsed by noxious ones. The person may no longer be able to interpret complex visual stimuli, but she can usually derive pleasure from looking at pictures and observing movement and color. She may no longer be able to understand complex speech, but music and other environmental sounds can enrich her sensory experience. Smell, touch, and taste require little interpretation in order to be fully appreciated. Therefore, an appropriate level of sensory stimulation is important.

Rhythm seems to be a sense that is retained for a long time. Even very impaired individuals brighten up and follow along well in activities with a strong rhythmic component, such as dancing, sawing wood, and threading beads. Motor-impaired clients can walk with more ease when a good rhythm is established and clients are better able to follow through with a task if simple repetitive instructions are given in a rhythmic tone.

Another important sense, and one rarely added to the basic five, is the sense of movement. This is the sensation of our body moving in space, such as swinging or rocking, and the feeling of our limbs moving in relation to the rest of our body. We are not usually conscious of this sense, although we do hear athletes and dancers speak of the "joy of movement." We observe it in children as they run, scamper, and climb. Lack of movement leads to muscle wasting and joint stiffness, and the immobile person may actually lose touch with her body. Movement and attention to the sensation of movement should be part of any complete activity program.

It is essential to guard against sensory overload. The person with AD has a limited capacity to process large amounts of stimulation and to sort out pertinent stimuli from extraneous background. Sensory experiences must be kept simple and direct. When a multisensory experience is being offered, all the senses involved should be directed at the same objective. Frequent and well-timed rest periods are also essential.

Emotions

The client may not always express her feelings appropriately, but they are real and require an outlet, especially when they are difficult to verbalize. Negative feelings such as anger and frustration may be dissipated through vigorous and aggressive physical activity. Pleasant emotions such as joy, tenderness, pride, and self-esteem can be expressed during sharing and caring sessions and life review. Animals and babies often evoke positive feelings in clients. The relationship is mutually unconditional and so poses no threat to either party. Sensory experiences can be stimulated through such things as fragrances and music,[2]

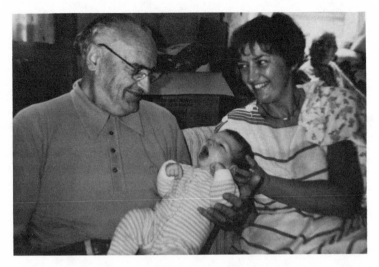

Babies have a way of communicating without words.

which often bring back feelings associated with an event in the past. Even though the memory of the event may have faded, the emotions linked with the sensation often remain and can be rekindled.

Remote Memory

Some clients seem to "live in the past," but appropriate recollection of past events, former accomplishments, and significant relationships can be very comforting to a client who is insecure in her present environment.[3] They provide pleasure, help reaffirm self-esteem, and provide a link with more stable times. Unrealistic attempts to resume or encourage activities at which the client had been very proficient, however, may cause frustration and engender a sense of despair as the client is vividly confronted with her failing skills. A realistic balance between pride in past accomplishments and expression of current competencies is important.

Perseveration

Although perseveration has been identified as a potential problem, the tendency to persist in repetitive behavior can be used positively. The client can be offered activities that are very repetitive in nature with little fear of her becoming bored. In fact, activities that involve many repetitions of one simple step seem to offer a certain comfort, as the need to make decisions, remember a sequence, and plan out the next step is eliminated.

4   Programing for the Clients' Needs

Why Do We Do the Things We Do, and Why Is It So Important to Keep Doing Them?

We have seen how the process of Alzheimer's disease limits the affected individual's ability to function. He often appears to have lost interest in activities, becomes socially withdrawn, and resists trying new activities. Despite this apparent lassitude, though, the person is often restless and agitated. He seems to feel a need to be active, to be involved.

Responsible programing should aim at giving the person with AD alternative means of fulfilling his personal needs. In order to understand these needs more clearly, we should look at them in a structured format.

A Hierarchy of Needs

Abraham Maslow referred to a hierarchy of needs.[1] At the base of this hierarchy are the physiological needs of food, clothing, and shelter. When these have been addressed, the need for security predominates. Higher up on the hierarchy are the individual's psychosocial needs: identity, control, autonomy, self-esteem, the esteem of others, inclusion, meaningful relationships, and meaningful communication. The basic needs of elderly persons, especially those who are dependent due to disability, must be carefully monitored.

Our concern in this discussion, however, is for security and the psychosocial needs, which remain vulnerable even when the basic physical needs are met.

The Need for Security

Few of us can function well unless we have a reasonable sense of security or safety. Memory loss, perceptual impairment, and inadequate communication skills make the AD client's world unpredictable and at times frightening. Fear of the future, disorientation, and spatial distortions can result in debilitating anxiety and even panic, which can seriously undermine his ability to cope. A calm, predictable and accepting environment can provide the sense of security that enables a client to make full use of his abilities.

Psychosocial Needs

Identity—the awareness of who one is and how one relates to others—is threatened as the person with AD withdraws from the activities that reinforce his self-awareness. Meaningful activities and accepting relationships can help reestablish a positive self-image and strengthen the client's sense of identity.

Control refers to our need to make an impact on our environment, that is, to move things in the direction of our own choosing. It may be as simple as watering a plant or as complex as running a multinational corporation. The person with AD is often at the mercy of an unpredictable environment. His efforts to control it are often unsuccessful. Helped to identify those tasks that they can do and provided with the supports that will ensure success, many clients can regain some sense of control.

Autonomy is control turned inward. It is the need to manage our own affairs and care for our own bodies independently. The entire process of maturation is a drive to autonomy. It is a need that is felt very strongly and one that cannot be surrendered without serious consequences to the individual's personal sense of well-being. The person who cannot go out unattended because he may become lost or who is no longer capable of dressing or bathing himself must still be given every possible opportunity to retain some independence. As simple an act as choosing the color of nail polish is an expression of autonomy.

Self-esteem and the esteem of others refer to one's appreciation of one's own personal value and one's perception of how one is valued by others. We judge ourselves by the quality of our achievements as measured against a standard, whether it be personal or absolute. Others judge us in the same way. The person whose skills are gradually diminishing is vulnerable to self-deprecation. Activities that project the client's strengths while minimizing his weaknesses can help to bolster self-esteem. An accepting and nonjudgmental environment can contribute, as well.

Inclusion—membership in a group and identification with a larger body—supports an individual's sense of identity and provides security. Membership in a group is usually maintained by active participation. A noncontributing member or one who behaves inappropriately is often excluded. Social isolation is one of the most painful losses associated with AD.

Meaningful communication and meaningful relationships go hand in hand, since relationships are bonded by communication. Communication can be either verbal or nonverbal. Language disturbances are probably among the most devastating effects of AD, in that they interfere with the client's capacity to interact with others on an abstract level.

Having identified these needs, we are better able to appreciate the significance of specific activities such as grooming, light chores, helping others, and group discussions as components of an activity program. All of these are the simple acts by which most of us express our psychosocial needs.

5   Designing a Program

Laying Down the Infrastructure

Program design determines the character of the physical
environment, the types of activities that will be part of the
program, the schedule and pace of activities, and the staffing requirements as they relate to specific events.

The Physical Environment

The physical environment in which the program is conducted must be given special attention. Since the person
with Alzheimer's disease is likely to have perceptual difficulties, the setting must address more than the basic
requirements of space, esthetic appeal, lighting, air circula-
tion, cleanliness, and accessibility—requirements that are
common to all programs. The area should be free of ambigu-
ities. It should be consistent and predictable. For example,
floor and wall areas should be distinct from each other.
Steps and other obstacles must be clearly visible. The floor
should be free of any markings that could be perceived as
obstacles by the perceptually impaired client. Furniture
should have clear limits and be distinct from its surroundings. Traffic areas must be free of any hidden obstacles such
as chair legs that extend out beyond the seat.

Contrasting colors can be used effectively to distinguish furniture from the surrounding area. In addition, color can be used to reinforce visual perspective in the room. If the floor and walls meld into one another, distances become very difficult to judge accurately.

Essential facilities, such as washrooms, should be visible from the program area and be clearly labeled. Some modern signing systems (such as the "Adam" and "Eve" signs that designate some restaurant washrooms) can be very confusing to the cognitively impaired person.

The space should be divided into areas that are permanently dedicated to specific activities: a work area for crafts and messy activities, a kitchen for meal preparation, a lounge area for relaxation, discussions, and teas, and a dining area for meals or small crafts. This permanent arrangement minimizes the need to move furniture and materials and maintains a consistent environment. It also reinforces the clients' routine of moving from one area to another.

There should be an easily cleared area available for gross motor activities such as exercises, dancing, and floor games. The area need not be permanently clear, since large open spaces often intimidate posturally insecure persons.

Attention must be paid to the quality and quantity of sensory stimuli in the environment. The area should include interesting focal objects, but it must not be overly stimulating. Although bright colors are good in moderation, the general ambiance of the setting should be subdued and neutral. Extraneous stimuli such as background noise and movement should be minimized. Soundproof barriers between activity areas are useful, providing they do not complicate the space that clients must negotiate to move from one area to another.

Well-marked exits are usually considered to be essential in any program facility. However, the sight of the exit may prompt the client with AD to wander off unobserved. A new client who is anxious in an unfamiliar setting may wish desperately to go home. The presence of an obvious exit may cause her to persist in trying to leave and make it difficult for the staff to help her settle down. Only one exit, which is easily monitored, should be left apparent. The others can be disguised by painting or papering them to match the wall. In order to avoid creating a closed-in feeling, and to disguise the door further, a mirror can be placed on it. It then appears to the clients to be an opened but impassable space.

Access to a long corridor or other safe walking area is useful for those clients who have a need to pace and work off restlessness. Many specialized facilities have built-in circular "walking corridors" for this purpose.

The program area should provide appropriate clues to help clients orient themselves as to place and time. These include clocks (preferably analog), large bank-style calendars, signs, and articles or decorations in keeping with the season or current holiday.

Familiar signs and symbols are much more meaningful than unfamiliar ones to the person with memory impairment. Which of the above do you think would be more meaningful?

The "Day Away" program area consists of one large room with an adjacent cloakroom and washroom. Specific activity areas are designated by furniture groupings. A space of approximately fifteen hundred square feet accommodates eight clients, two staff members, and four or five volunteers. Clients and their helpers are able to disperse into small groups with a minimum of conflict and interference. The area could be improved with the addition of a separate yet easily monitored space for those clients who need to go off and be alone every now and then.

The location of the program within the community is also an important consideration. "Day Away" is housed within a large community health complex that also includes an extended care facility. Fortunately, access to the program area leads through the out-patient family health clinic and past a senior citizens' center. Consequently, the clients usually encounter healthy persons when they enter and leave the program, and any feeling they have of coming to a medical facility is minimized.

Selecting Meaningful Activities

Once the environment has been arranged, appropriate activities should be identified. For an activity to be meaningful to a client, it must meet certain important criteria. The activity must have relevance to the client, be voluntary, and offer the client a reasonable chance for success. It must in some way address the client's personal psychosocial needs, and its purpose must be obvious to the client.

An activity that does not relate positively to the client's social, intellectual, and emotional status will not be meaningful and may, in fact, be interpreted as an affront. The activity should never be (or be perceived by the client to be) demeaning, childish, or in any way threatening to her self-esteem.

Although clients may be encouraged or even coerced into overcoming inertia or anxiety, they should not be forced to participate in any program activity that they continue to resist. The benefits of participation will likely be exceeded by the negative feelings aroused.

The success of an activity should be measured by the client's standards as well as by the standards of others. No amount of praise will cause a person to feel gratified by a product that is below her established standards. In order to ensure success, achievement in the activity must be within the client's physical, intellectual, and perceptual abilities.

This requires an accurate assessment of the client's skills and an accurate analysis of the task requirements.

To determine whether an activity can offer the client an opportunity to meet her psychosocial needs, we must first identify the particular needs that are important to that client. Then we analyze the activity for its potential to address that need. Some examples are: manicure, make-up, or hairdressing for the lady who has a poor self-image; inclusion in a group project for a gentleman who is socially isolated.

Every activity should have a purpose that is obvious to the client. "Busy work" is demeaning. It is also difficult to commit oneself to an activity that has no particular goal. Some activities may be done just for fun, but most projects must have a clear purpose. Sometimes the purpose is self-evident, such as grooming or cleaning up. Still, for some clients, reinforcement of the purpose may be necessary; this may be accomplished by repeating the activity on a small scale—for example, combing hair and freshening make-up before going home. At other times the purpose must be built into the project; for example, the outlet for crafts can be well established before construction begins: articles can be made for sale at a bazaar or as gifts for a grandchild. This approach helps ensure a high standard of production and makes some activities, such as stenciling or making pom-poms, more acceptable to clients who might otherwise perceive them as childish. It also adds a spark of interest to the project and supports a sense of communality. Cooking and baking projects are ideal, since the products can be enjoyed by the clients immediately. If a client is participating in a group effort, she should be kept informed of her personal contribution. This may require frequent repetition, but the effort is well worth the interest and enthusiasm it generates.

When a suitable activity has been identified, it must be adapted to match the capacities of the clients. This involves two basic exercises: grading activities and analyzing activities.

Grading Activities

Grading activities refers to increasing or decreasing the demands an activity places on the participant. A simple example would be a gradual increase in the weight that a body builder lifts. There are many ways in which activities

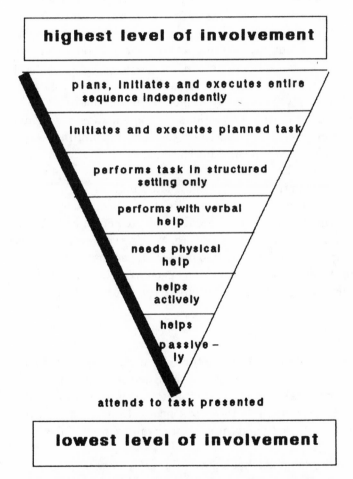

highest level of involvement

plans, initiates and executes entire sequence independently

initiates and executes planned task

performs task in structured setting only

performs with verbal help

needs physical help

helps actively

helps passively

attends to task presented

lowest level of involvement

Activities may be graded in a variety of ways. One very effective way is to vary the degree of involvement by the client in planning, initiating, and executing a task.

can be graded. One of the most effective ways is to vary the degree of involvement on the part of the client. In making muffins, for example, total involvement would mean planning, organizing, sequencing, and executing the entire operation. If this requires some skills that the client does not have, she may still be able to mix premeasured ingredients and continue from there, or she may only be able to pour premixed batter into the muffin tin or to hold the muffin tin while someone else pours the batter. The tin may not need to be held, but physical contact with the activity may keep her attention. (Occasionally a more astute client will object to "artificial" involvement, and thus it should be suggested with sensitivity and only when the client is not likely to have overt or covert objections.) In some instances a client may only be able to watch someone making muffins, keep company, smell the muffins baking, and then pass judgment on the finished product. Even at this limited level, she is involved in the process of muffin making!

Activities that are most suitable for this kind of grading are those that involve several steps, each of which is fairly simple and repetitive in nature. Making spaghetti sauce is a good example. There are so many things that must be chopped and stirred that many people can be involved to various degrees and contribute to the communal effort.

Analyzing Activities

Activities are analyzed by three basic parameters: the physical, perceptual, sensory, and cognitive demands that the activity makes on the participant; the value of the activity to the participant in terms of sensory stimulation and satisfaction of needs; and the success or failure potential of the activity.

The demands that a particular activity will make on a client can be determined by breaking the activity down into its individual steps and by reviewing each step in terms of the following questions:

- What physical abilities does the activity demand? How

much strength, endurance, coordination, flexibility, and dexterity must the participant have in order to perform the activity successfully and in comfort?

- What kind of sensory acuity is required? To what extent must the participant be able to see, hear, feel, or balance in order to succeed?
- What kind of perceptual processes are involved in this activity? Must the person have good body awareness? Is the accurate perception of space and spatial relations important? Must she be able to perceive shape, size, and color accurately? How important is eye-hand coordination?
- What cognitive functions are necessary? Will the participant be required to make decisions, anticipate and solve problems, make calculations, organize and sequence, make judgments? How critical is the accuracy of these judgments? Must the participant be able to remember, express herself verbally, and call upon factual knowledge? To what extent will the participant be able to call upon overlearned patterns of movement? Will this task require new learning? What intensity of attention and duration of attention span are required by this activity to ensure a successful outcome?

The value that an activity may have for a client can be determined by analyzing the activity in terms of its potential to satisfy the psychosocial needs we have previously discussed: identity, self-esteem, esteem of others, autonomy, control, meaningful communication, meaningful relationships, and inclusion. A review of the sensory stimulation that is available to a client as a result of her participation in an activity is also important; stimulation can be visual, in terms of movement, color, and patterns; tactile, in terms of texture, pressure, and temperature; and proprioceptive, which refers to the sense of movement of one's own body. The sounds, tastes, and smells that are associated with the activity should also be considered.

Our experience at "Day Away" suggests that the most successful activities are those that are highly repetitive.

They permit the clients to establish a rhythm and a sense of competence and continuity, and the clients needn't worry about the next step. We have found that the most successful and enjoyable activities also have a very broad range of successful outcomes, so the potential for failure is virtually eliminated. It is impossible to sand a block of wood for a cutting board badly: the more you rub, the better it becomes.

Scheduling and Routine

Once appropriate activities have been determined, they must be put into a time frame. A schedule that accommodates fluctuations in the clients' energy levels is important. Once the schedule has been established, it should be adhered to, as the clients will find comfort in its predictability and consistency.

Although allowances must be made for differences among individuals, the energy level of persons with AD is usually higher at the beginning of the day. Consequently, it is best to have the most demanding and structured activities in the morning. The schedule that is used at "Day Away" is outlined at the end of this chapter.

The duration of each activity is another matter to consider. It is important to observe the reaction of clients individually and as a group, but, in general, structured, nondemanding activities such as simple crafts, grooming, sing-alongs, or floor games (like beanbag toss) are enjoyed for a considerable amount of time. It seems to take the clients some time to get into the swing of the activity, but once the pattern is established, they are loath to leave it. Unstructured times, such as freewheeling discussions or rest periods, seem to be tolerated for no more than half an hour.

Staffing

The staff-to-client ratio at "Day Away" is usually two staff members and four volunteers to seven or eight clients. Staffing requirements at any one time in the program, however, will depend on the nature of the activity taking place. When a new activity is being introduced, it is essential to have a one-to-one ratio. This helps ensure success in the activity on the first try. It also gives the staff an opportunity to make valuable observations about the clients' abilities and reactions and to determine how much supervision each client will require in the future. Structured group activities, such as meals or group discussions, are best staffed at a minimum. Two or three members of the staff should be sufficient for eight clients. During these times, large numbers of staff would tend to overwhelm the clients and so reduce their independence. Staff and volunteers who are not directly involved usually withdraw but remain available to help clients who need individual attention or who must leave the group.

Many of the processes described in this chapter are followed intuitively by persons accustomed to working with the handicapped, and many successful programs have been developed that do not accord attention to the specific items outlined here. Nonetheless, a review of the practices of a program in relation to these elements can be useful in validating and reinforcing existing practices as well as in identifying areas that require more attention.

A Schedule of Daily Activities

08:15. Van Pick-up Begins Route with One Staff Member on Board

Objective: Reinforce the clients' awareness of their destination and make their trip to the day center as comfortable and secure as possible.

The staff member meets each client at her door. The sight of a familiar face reassures the client and reinforces the feeling that her presence at the program is appreciated.

09:00. Arrival and Orientation

Objective: Ensure relaxed entry into the program and reaffirm place, time, purpose, and person.

Clients are welcomed by the staff. They are shown where to hang their clothes. If clients need help with removal of clothing, help is given in such a way as to encourage participation, not dependence, from the client. Introductions and greetings are conducted in the lounge area, and clients are given their name tags. Coffee or tea may be served to reinforce the social nature of the gathering. The orientation calendar is reviewed to reaffirm place and time. Appropriate seasonal materials are presented and discussed. Plans for the day are reviewed. If a craft or a special event is planned, it is discussed and demonstrated briefly.

10:00. Activities

Objective: Provide meaningful activity and sensory stimulation relevant to the client's level of ability.

These may be crafts or other specially planned activities. Each client's participation has been planned beforehand. Materials and equipment are prepared and set out in the appropriate area. Each client is invited to move to the designated area and is briefly told what she will be doing there. Explanations relate to the prior group discussion of the activity.

11:00. Snack

Objective: Reinforce social skills and social contacts. Encourage fluid and nutritional intake.

Clients who have finished their activity prepare the snack and set the table. If the activity was baking, the baked goods are served at this time. Pleasant table manners and conversation are encouraged. Photographs of past events may be circulated to encourage conversation. Clients are encouraged to bring in mementos that can be presented to the group at this time.

11:30. Exercise Period

Objective: Maintain strength, range of motion, and body awareness. Reinforce socialization with dancing.

Clients participate in a course of mobility and strengthening exercises. One-on-one guidance is given to those clients who cannot follow independently. The session concludes with a short dance period with familiar music.

12:00. Meal Preparation

Objective: Maintain independent living skills.

Meal preparation tasks such as setting the table, making fruit salad, preparing a soup mix, are broken down and assigned to clients according to their skills and interests.

12:30. Lunch

Objective: Maintain eating skills and nutrition.

A full-course meal is provided in order to free the caregiver from cooking on that day and to give the staff an opportunity to try some problem-solving techniques with clients who are having difficulties managing mealtimes at home. Staff members eat with the clients to act as models and to stimulate appropriate behavior at the table.

13:00. Clean-up

Objective: Maintain independent living skills.

Clients clear the table and wash the dishes.

13:30. Grooming

Objective: Maintain self-care skills and positive self-awareness.

Clients are encouraged to use the washroom, comb their hair, reapply make-up, and generally tidy up. Manicures are done at this time. Clients who are potentially incontinent are brought to the washroom at regular two-hour intervals.

13:45. Gross Motor Activity

Objective: Provide appropriate gross motor activity and social interaction.

This may be a walk outdoors (in good weather) or floor games, such as beanbag toss and horseshoes.

14:15. Wind-down

Objective: Review day's events, reaffirm group membership, and prepare for departure.

This usually includes a sing-along accompanied by the serving of juice. The day ends with a review of the day's activities and accomplishments. Clients are removed individually toward the end to dress for departure.

15:00. Van Departure with One Staff Member on Board

Objective: Ensure that clients remain secure in the knowledge that they will arrive home safely.

The schedule remains flexible to accommodate individual client's needs and interests. After lunch, one client may wish to return to a craft she enjoyed. Another may enjoy doing some light housekeeping instead of participating in a structured activity.

Seasonal events and outings are scheduled throughout the year and form a large part of the program. Picnics, outings to pick fruit, and bus excursions are examples.

6 Activities

This chapter describes a variety of activities that persons with AD may take part in. The rationale for each activity is also described.

Exercise

The aims of the daily exercise period are
- to maintain muscle strength
- to maintain joint flexibility
- to provide a gentle cardiopulmonary workout
- to help clients maintain body awareness through the sensation of movement
- to provide a pleasurable experience and a sense of competence in being able to follow along with the group and move freely

The exercise leader provides simple, rhythmic instructions. The same words are used each time, and the exercise routine is presented in the same order each day. (A sample exercise program is presented at the end of this section.) The routine also includes a dance session, which the clients enjoy very much. Big band music is a favorite. Clients' participation is facilitated by the rhythmic sounds of a vibraphone or appropriate music when it is available.

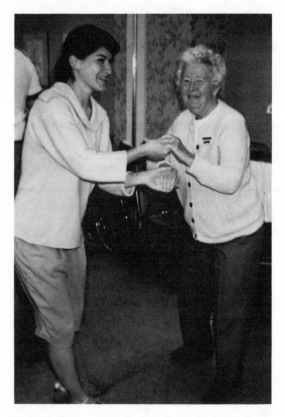

Dancing to an old-time favorite brings out the good spirit in everyone

Clients who have difficulty following the exercise routine are given one-on-one help. When one-on-one assistance is being offered, it is especially important for the helper to remain aware of the objectives of this activity. As long as the client is moving in response to the leader's instructions and is content with his performance, all the aims of the session are being met, and the quality and accuracy of his movements are of secondary importance. Moreover, it is questionable whether an effort to encourage more accurate movements would be of value. The interference of the helper may distract the client, compromise his sense of competence, and limit his enjoyment of the exercise. On the other hand, a client who is perplexed and unable to perform to his own satisfaction needs help.

Guidance is provided in as unobtrusive a fashion as possible, applying the techniques of manual assistance that are outlined in detail in chapter 7. Generally, verbal direction to individual clients from their helpers is kept at a minimum, since it tends to interfere with the instructions of the leader and could be disruptive to the rest of the group.

Exercise Program

1. Warm-ups (Seated)
   - a. Head and neck   chin to chest, return ×5
     turn to right, center, left ×10
     tilt to right ×3
     tilt to left ×3
   - b. Shoulders   shrug both shoulders ×10
     right only ×5
     left only ×5
   - c. Elbows   hands to shoulders, relax ×10
   - d. Hands   make fist, relax, stretch, relax ×10
   - e. Hips   raise one foot slightly, down ×10
     raise other foot, down ×10
   - f. Knees   straighten one leg, down ×10
     straighten other leg, down ×10
   - g. Feet   heels up, down ×10
     toes up, down ×10

2. Active Exercise (Standing, Use Chair for Balance if Needed)
   - a. Shoulders   hands to shoulders, reach up, hands to shoulders ×10
   - b. Waist   hands on hips, twist to right, center, left, center ×10
   - c. Waist   hands on hips, stretch to left, center, right, center ×10
   - d. Knees   slight knee bends ×10

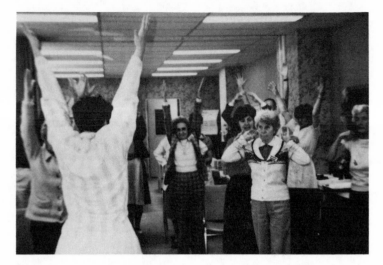

The exercise group: precision is not important, movement is.

    e. Hips   knees straight, kick one leg ×10
                       kick other leg ×10
    f. Balance   hands on hips, sway side to side ×10

3. Dance to Music

4. Cool Down
    a. Swing arms slowly
    b. Roll head gently
    c. Face—tighten, make a face, relax ×3, breathe
    d. Knees—press together, relax ×3, breathe
    e. Feet and hands—tighten, relax ×3*

Other Gross Motor Activities

For many clients, a surplus of physical energy with no meaningful outlet may result in restlessness and, sometimes, agitation. Therefore, regular gross motor activities are an essential part of the daily plan.

*The original exercise program used at "Day Away" was designed by Anne Opzoomer O.T. (C).

Walks outside in fine weather are usually well received. The group can walk out to the playground to watch children or stroll through the neighborhood just to keep in touch with the community. Staff members can draw clients' attention to significant sights, sounds, and aromas while they are out.

Organized gross motor activities, such as games, are sometimes awkward to introduce to adults who may be sensitive about seemingly childish activities; however, sometimes these games arise spontaneously. A staff member may pick up a beanbag and jokingly toss it to a client. The client catches it and tosses it back. Another client is drawn into the game and, before realizing it, everyone is involved in a rousing game of toss and catch. It is much easier to initiate such an activity in an informal way, because that does not threaten anyone's self-esteem and participation remains spontaneous and voluntary.

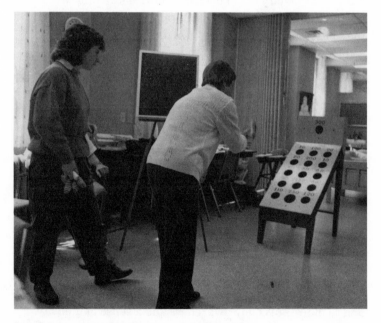

Beanbag toss is a favorite gross motor activity.

Beanbag toss, set up in a minitournament fashion, with a scoreboard and teams, can be very successful. The tournament format, with clients taking their turns, playing by the rules, and recording the scores, gives the game a structure to which clients can relate comfortably. Conversely, informal "hacking around" may confuse and make uncomfortable those clients who cannot follow the jokes. Some of the more apraxic clients may need to have the action of tossing the beanbag at the target modeled for them, but in five trials, almost every client can succeed in getting a score on the board.

Some complex games must be modified and simplified. Lawn croquet, the rules of which can boggle the mind of even the most astute, can be modified into a simple target game. Two pins are set out to make a goal. Clients take turns knocking the ball between the goal posts. The number of trials needed to get the ball between the goal posts is counted, and the lowest team score wins. We had an example of the tenacity of old behavior patterns during this game. A lady who had been an avid golfer persisted in trying to use the croquet mallet as a driver. A croquet ball struck with the force she intended to use would have been dangerous. Efforts to teach her the proper croquet stroke only resulted in frustration, but the game was saved when she was convinced that she could putt the ball nicely between the posts.

Bowling and shuffleboard are other games that accommodate well the abilities of AD clients. The common elements in all these games are that the objective is obvious, the results are immediately apparent to the participants, and it is acceptable for adults to play them.

Grooming and Hygiene

Attention to grooming and personal hygiene helps to build self-esteem. It keeps clients in touch with their appearance and so maintains body awareness and a sense of identity. Activities include hair and skin care, oral hygiene and denture care, manicures, and make-up. Ladies are encouraged to experiment with colors of nail polish, lipstick, and eyeshadow. Samplers of perfume and cologne are available, also.

All clients are encouraged to be as independent as possible. For sanitary reasons, all make-ups must be applied with disposable applicators. Unfortunately, this sometimes makes it difficult for ladies who are accustomed to using their own articles and to having a personal routine. Those who need to have things done for them are involved by watching in the mirror and by selecting the shades they prefer. The psychosocial need for control is addressed in this way.

Female AD clients generally look forward to these sessions; they enjoy the lift a new hairdo or a fresh manicure brings. This is also an intimate social time, a time for sharing and caring on a very personal level.

Special attention to the personal hygiene of the person with AD is of particular importance. As the person loses the ability to do many of the routine self-care tasks, not only may his appearance deteriorate but his general health may suffer, as well. Improper skin care may lead to skin breakdown. Poor oral hygiene may cause dental problems, restricting the person's ability to eat comfortably and, therefore, interfering with nutrition.

Family members often find it difficult to become involved in these intimate areas. When these activities are routinely included in the program, staff members are able to identify problems, bring them to the attention of the caregiver, and offer techniques and suggestions for coping with them at home.

A regular toileting routine is essential for clients who have had difficulty with continence. Bladder accidents often occur because the client has "forgotten" to attend to the message from a full bladder or, having responded to the urge to void, had difficulty initiating a trip to the washroom before it was too late. Once in the washroom, the client may have difficulty managing his clothing, and the frustration

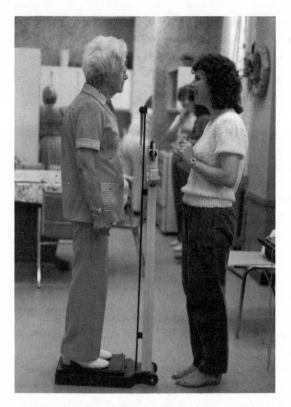

Health monitoring includes taking regular measurements of
weight and blood pressure.

and delay may cause an accident. Those clients who have a
history of incontinence are generally accompanied to the
washroom by staff members who can identify the source of
the problem, introduce the appropriate helping techniques,
and relate these techniques to family members. In this way,
the incidence of accidents at home can also be reduced.
Appropriate times for reminding these clients to go to the
washroom are built into the program routine; for example,
between activities, after meals, before going out for a walk,
and before going home.

Routine attention to the clients' personal hygiene by

program staff also facilitates the introduction of health monitoring by the nurse in the program. On accompanying a client to the washroom, a staff member may notice a client's discomfort on voiding. Since a client with memory loss may not remember to mention such pain to anyone after the fact, a urinary tract infection could go unnoticed until it has led to other complications. Many clients do not localize pain or perceive pain accurately. Staff members giving manicures or attending to other areas of the clients' personal hygiene and grooming may notice burned fingers, cuts, or bruises and can alert families to possible hazards in the home.

Times for Socializing

Although social interaction is encouraged throughout most activities, certain activities are planned especially to stimulate socialization.

Orientation time at the beginning of the day is intended to confirm time, place, and membership in the group. Group members contribute to the discussion of a current theme or topic at their own level of comfort and prepare for the events of the day.

Coffee break is aimed at giving clients an opportunity to practice well-maintained social skills and to participate in self-directed social interchange.

Sing-along is another time for clients to contribute to a group effort, each at his own level of ability. Camaraderie, engendered by music and familiar melodies, reinforces group feeling and addresses the clients' need for inclusion.

Wind-down at the end of the day consists of a review of the day's activities. Each client's achievements are highlighted, and individual contributions to the day's events are identified.

Communication skills are at the heart of any social interaction. The individual with impaired language skills can be painfully isolated unless those around him employ thoughtful and insightful communication techniques.

Learning how to wait is essential. Many clients are slow to respond and have difficulty keeping pace with conversations unless others make a point of slowing down.

Spoken language is often understood more easily by clients when it is accompanied by visual prompts and cues. Staff members should try to include props when discussing themes during orientation. For this reason, too, nonverbal communication is important as an accompaniment and supplement to the spoken word. Facial expression and body language can confirm or negate what is said, depending on whether or not they are consistent with the ideas being expressed.

Above all, the client needs to know that he is safe and accepted, no matter what he says or how it comes out. Paraphasias and disinhibition can result in socially embarrassing situations for the client unless an accepting, nonjudgmental atmosphere is maintained.

Memory loss can expose the client to unsettling and embarrassing situations that threaten his security. Open-ended, direct questions, no matter how friendly or well meaning, can be very threatening to the client who cannot remember. Volunteers should be discouraged from asking clients for specific information unless they are sure that the client can answer comfortably.

The acceptance and appreciation that clients develop for one another is probably the single most valuable benefit of a day program. In their zeal to provide a structured, active program, staff members must not overlook or impede the development of relationships between clients.

Housekeeping and Meal Preparation

Tasks at which the client was proficient in the past take on a new importance as the ability to meet new challenges is lost. Washing and drying dishes, sweeping, tidying, and dusting are significant contributions to the program and are genuinely appreciated. They are important at a time when the clients' opportunities to help and to accept thanks are limited. In fact, volunteers quickly learn to curb their impulse to wash the dishes. They realize that simple but essential jobs such as this are reserved for clients who have a special need to be helpful. Having identified these competencies in a client at the program, the staff can pass this information on to the family members and suggest that these tasks be reserved for the client at home.

Jobs that require a number of short steps, such as setting the table, are best broken down into individual components. The client is given the place mats and is asked to put them all out first. He then places a napkin at each setting. This is followed by the glasses, forks, spoons, and so on. He then fills all the glasses with ice water. In this way, a comfortable, repetitive pattern is established, and the client can proceed with confidence through each step.

One-step jobs such as feeding fish or watering a plant provide the client with little opportunity to practice and develop a sense of competence before the job is finished. It often leaves him feeling dissatisfied and not quite sure whether he has accomplished the objective. Polishing furniture, however, is a job that can be demonstrated and practiced and still leaves plenty of polishing to do once the client has the idea.

The facility's kitchen can be expected to get heavy use. Each day clients can prepare dessert, soup, and snacks for the program. Picnics and outings in summer provide a reason for clients to prepare sandwiches, fresh vegetables, and muffins or snacking cakes. Occasionally, special meals are prepared for particular purposes. The clients at "Day Away" prepared huge amounts of spaghetti sauce for a fundraising dinner. On another occasion, they made a large pot of chili for a staff member to save him the chore of cooking while his wife was in the hospital having their second child.

Recipes that AD clients prepare most successfully are those that lend themselves to an "assembly-line" organization and that do not require precise proportions of ingredients. The following are examples of such recipes.

Chili

INGREDIENTS
ground beef (enough to be stirred comfortably in a large pot)
chopped onions (as much as one client can chop while the
   ground beef is being browned)
chopped celery
chopped green pepper
grated carrots
olive oil to sauté vegetables
one large can of tomato sauce
canned kidney beans (enough to fill the pot, leaving room to
   stir occasionally)
chili powder (to taste, adding one teaspoonful at a time)

EQUIPMENT
one large stew pot
wooden mixing spoon
can opener
cutting boards
paring knives
grater
platter or shallow bowl to grate carrots into

METHOD
   Set up work stations. Have separate cutting boards,
knives, and vegetables to be chopped at each place. Have
the pot and other necessary items such as the meat, a stirring spoon, a can opener, and the cans arranged near the
stove.
   Assemble examples of all ingredients and present them
to the group along with a discussion of the dish to be prepared and the purpose for preparing it.
   Identify the individual jobs to be done and elicit volunteers, if appropriate, for each job. It is best to direct a client
toward jobs that are suited to his particular level of ability.
For example, a client who is capable of following step-by-
step instructions or who can take initiative in a multistep
task is more likely to feel comfortable opening the cans,
draining the beans, and adding individual ingredients to

the pot, while someone less capable will be more comfortable with a repetitive job such as chopping the celery.

Each client is directed to his work area. Four clients may work around the table, chopping vegetables, while one goes to the stove to brown the meat, drain off the fat, and sauté the chopped vegetables in olive oil.

Another client may open the cans and add the contents, along with other ingredients, to the pot.

As each job is finished, clients move to another area to relax or to take over another step in the process.

Finally, the pot is left to simmer while the aroma of chili fills the room and drifts down the corridor.

Everyone is invited to sample the product when it is cooked.

Spaghetti Sauce

INGREDIENTS
ground beef
chopped onions
chopped celery
chopped green and/or red pepper
grated carrots
olive oil to sauté vegetables
canned tomato sauce to fill the pot
one can of tomato paste for each can of tomato sauce used
basil, oregano, hot peppers, salt, and garlic powder to taste.

EQUIPMENT
one large stew pot
wooden mixing spoon
can opener
cutting boards
paring knives
grater
platter or shallow bowl to grate carrots into

METHOD
Same as for chili.

Cheese Scones

INGREDIENTS
2 cups biscuit mix
½ cup milk
grated cheese (quantity is not important)
flour for dusting table while rolling and cutting dough

EQUIPMENT
measuring cup
mixing bowl
mixing spoon
grater and platter
small cookie cutters
cookie sheet
rolling pins

METHOD

Set up a work area with a large mixing bowl, a mixing spoon, and premeasured milk and biscuit mix.

Set up another work area with the cheese, a grater, and a platter.

Set up two or three work areas with rolling pins and small cookie cutters.

One client mixes the dough while another grates the cheese.

Knead the cheese into the dough.

Divide the dough into two or three portions, depending on how many clients will be rolling and cutting biscuits.

Each client rolls out his portion of the dough on a lightly floured table and cuts out small biscuits. Very small cutters offer the client a chance for more repetitions of a familiar and comfortable task. They also make dainty snacks for coffee time.

Biscuits are arranged on an ungreased cookie sheet and baked according to package directions, taking into account shorter baking time for small biscuits.

This recipe can be altered by using apple juice instead of milk and adding chopped apples, sugar, and cinnamon.

Apple Tarts

INGREDIENTS
bulk recipe for pie pastry on Tenderflake container (This
    recipe is not sensitive to being overworked, as are
    conventional pie crust pastries.)
flour for dusting rolling surface
apples
sugar to taste
lemon juice
cornstarch or flour to thicken
butter to dot tops of tarts
cinnamon and nutmeg

METHOD
Set up one or two work stations with rolling pins, individual tart tins, a round cutter to cut tart shells, and flour to
dust the rolling surface.

Set up several work stations with cutting boards, paring
knives, and apples.

Set up one work area with a large mixing bowl, a mixing
spoon, sugar, cornstarch or flour, cinnamon, and lemon
juice.

One or two clients roll and cut pastry and line tart tins.

Several clients pare and chop apples.

Another client mixes chopped apples with remaining
ingredients and fills pastry shells.

One client decorates tops of tarts with pastry scraps and
dots them with butter.

Bake until pastry is golden brown and apples are tender.

Leftover tart filling can be cooked into apple sauce.

Apple Sauce, Jams, Fruit Salad

All of these foods lend themselves to the approach described
above. We have found that the clients enjoy the communal
"work bee" atmosphere. When the stress of organizing and
planning the entire project is removed, they can take the
opportunity to chat and joke while working.

Crafts

Crafts pose a special challenge to the activity programmer. Their appeal usually lies in their novelty and creativity. These are qualities that are not compatible with the abilities of most clients with AD. Nonetheless, there is much satisfaction to be gained from producing an article that has this type of appeal. If crafts are selected judiciously and are modified to accommodate the limited abilities of AD clients, they can be a very satisfying component of the program.

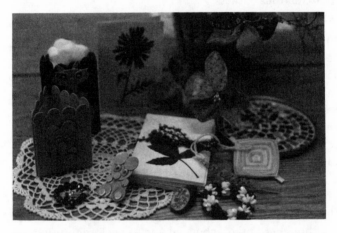

Some of the craft projects clients can make for sale at a local bazaar.

Crafts that are most successful with clients satisfy the following criteria:
- They are amenable to being broken down into individual steps that can be repeated frequently and with reasonable independence and competence on the part of the client.
- They produce a product that is pleasing to adults.
- Meaningful disposal or use of the product is assured.
- They have a low potential for failure, despite faulty judgment and/or dexterity on the part of the client.

- There is a pleasurable sensory experience inherent in each step of the task.

The following craft activities are generally well received by persons with Alzheimer's disease.

Wood Plaque Refrigerator Magnets, Brooches, and Key-Chains

Objective: Produce novelties to sell for fundraising or to give as gifts. These articles sell very well, and clients relate positively to this objective.

MATERIALS
pressed leaves and flowers (collected and dried during the summer)
Podgy clear acrylic sealer, glue, and fixative diluted with an equal amount of water
straight, knot-free branches of fragrant wood such as cedar, pine, etc., with a pleasing bark, between 1 and 1½ inches in diameter
small round magnets and/or
pin findings and/or
key-chain findings
fine-grained sandpaper
craft paper to cover the table to protect it in case of spills
(Using newspapers is not recommended, as the printed surface is distracting and makes it difficult for some clients to focus attention on their work. A clean, white surface is desirable.)

EQUIPMENT
miter box
light cross-cut saw
2 or 3 C-clamps
small paintbrushes

METHOD

Task 1: Cut Plaques

Clamp branch into miter box and clamp miter box onto a firm surface. With this set-up, one client can cut diagonal slices, about half an inch thick, from the branch. In order for all the slices to be even, the client may need to have a helper whose job is to move the branch along after each cut.

Sawing is a simple, familiar activity that establishes a comfortable rhythm and produces pleasing feedback for the worker. The aroma of the fresh wood being cut is also very pleasant.

Task 2: Sand Plaques

Tape one piece of fine sandpaper to the table for each client who will be participating. Clients are shown how to rub the cut surface of the plaque on the sandpaper until a smooth surface is achieved.

This set-up is appropriate for less able clients. The sanding process, again, is a simple, repetitive task. Performed in a group, sanding creates a "work bee" atmosphere. Because it demands little concentration on the part of the clients, they can chat while working comfortably. The aroma of the wood adds to the pleasant atmosphere. Most clients are able to judge the smoothness of the surface they are working on and so can appraise their own work. This is important in maintaining a sense of competence and independence.

Task 3: Decorate Plaques

Covering the table with craft paper, set up a work station for each client with a pot of diluted Podgy, a small paintbrush, and a selection of small pressed flowers and leaves.

The client selects a flower or leaf that will fit well onto the plaque and decides on a pleasing arrangement (simple arrangements are most effective).

The flower is then set aside and the client applies a base coat of Podgy to the more attractive surface of the plaque. Podgy goes on white but dries clear, so there is no need to worry about going over the edges. Because the Podgy is diluted, there is no need to be concerned about putting on too much. The task is virtually "failure-proof."

The flower is then arranged on the wet Podgy surface. It can be moved around quite easily with a toothpick before the Podgy dries. Many of these little plaques can be made and set aside for drying.

Task 4: Apply Finishing Coats

Set up work stations with craft paper on the table, pots of diluted Podgy, and a paintbrush for each client.

A coat of diluted Podgy is applied to each decorated plaque, which is then set aside to dry.

This process is repeated until a smooth finish is obtained.

The more coats, the better. Again, there is no potential for failure. Demands for attentiveness on the part of the clients are minimal, freeing them to interact among themselves as they are working. Podgy dries quite quickly, so several coats can be applied to each plaque during one activity session. Clean-up is easy because Podgy brushes wash up with water.

Task 5: Attach Findings

A magnet or a pin finding is glued to the back of each plaque.

To make a key-chain, clamp the finished plaque to a firm surface and set a small hole in one end using a nail and a hammer. A client can then drill a small hole using a hand drill.

Thread the plaque onto the key-chain finding.

Bookmarks

Objective: Produce novelties to sell at a bazaar for fundraising. These sell very well.

pressed leaves and flowers
exposed X-ray film, cut into oblongs 2 inches by 5 inches
Podgy sealer diluted with an equal amount of water
craft paper to cover the table

EQUIPMENT
small paintbrushes

METHOD
Same as for wood plaques.

This activity, too, is failure-proof. The clients enjoy looking through and selecting the pressed flowers. The activity
goes very quickly, which is probably one of its attractions,
since each bookmark is a new adventure. The product is sur-
prisingly elegant!

The planner would be wise to amass a very large stock of
pressed flowers during the summer and to enlist friends and
neighbors to cut and press flowers, as well. It would be a
lovely reminder of summer to work with flowers during the
winter months—if stocks could be made to last that long!
Autumn leaves make a nice seasonal change, too.

Hasty Notes

Objective: Produce novelties to sell for fundraising or to give
as gifts.

MATERIALS
fine-quality bond paper, letter sized
pressed leaves and flowers
Podgy sealer diluted with an equal amount of water
craft paper to cover the table
thin ribbon

EQUIPMENT
small paintbrushes
1 iron
2 clean tea towels

METHOD

Task 1: Fold Cards

Clients with fairly good fine-motor control and ability to appraise accuracy fold paper sheets into fourths and pass them to the group, who will decorate them.

Task 2: Decorate Cards

Set up work stations with craft paper on the table, pots of diluted Podgy, pressed flowers and leaves, and a paintbrush for each client.

The client takes a folded card, selects flowers, and decides on the arrangement.

The flowers are set aside, and the client applies a thin coat of diluted Podgy to the area where the flower arrangement will be placed.

The client arranges the flowers on the wet paper and applies another thin coat of diluted Podgy, taking care to dab down the tips of leaves and flowers.

The card is set aside to dry. No additional coats of Podgy are required.

This activity is a little more demanding in terms of accuracy and judgment on the part of the client. The flowers are not easily moved once they have been placed. It also requires a more delicate touch in applying the top coat of sealer.

Task 3: Iron Cards to Flatten Them

This task is appropriate for one client with a helper. Each card is placed between the two tea towels and is ironed with an iron on a medium setting.

The process of ironing is familiar and comfortable to most clients. Supervision is required for safety reasons and to help with the placement of the cards between the towels. This is a nice opportunity for a one-on-one session between the client and the helper.

Task 4: Tie Up Packages of Notes

Packages of six notes are tied together with a premeasured length of thin ribbon. A less capable client can participate by placing his finger on the knot while a helper or a more capable client ties the bow.

Stenciled Notes

Using commercially available seasonal stencils and colored markers or paint-dipped sponges, clients can stencil designs onto hasty notes. To ensure accuracy, each stencil is secured to the notepaper with four paper clips. The notes are folded, ironed, and packaged as above.

Woodwork

Any program fortunate enough to receive a donation of scraps of fine woods from a local furniture manufacturer or woodworker can make good use of them. Many of the people

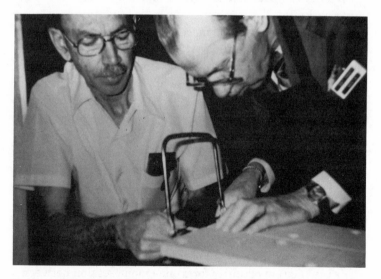

Feeling in control with a familiar job. This gentleman is cutting the pegs for a Hi-Q game.

in the program will enjoy sorting through them, identifying the various grains, appreciating the beauty of the wood, and recalling projects they made in the past. Cutting boards can be made from precut pieces of hardwood which clients sand down to a smooth finish and oil. Wood scraps with interesting knots and irregular shapes can be sanded and decorated with decoupage or dried flowers to make novelty wall plaques. The fragrance and texture of the material is particularly pleasant.

One gentleman in the "Day Away" program made several Hi-Q games for his grandchildren. He marked each hole through a template made from old X-ray film. Then he set each hole with a nail and hammer. Because it would have been difficult for him to drill each hole uniformly, he drilled all the holes right through the piece of wood and then glued a thinner piece of wood onto the bottom. The work was sealed with shellac, and then sanded and oiled to a fine finish. The pegs were cut from a piece of dowelling and sanded smooth. The project provided him with continuity and something of his own to look forward to each time he came to the program.

Work-oriented Activities

There are many jobs associated with the running of a program which clients are happy to help with, especially clients who are not particularly interested in crafts or housekeeping activities.

At "Day Away," the daily notes are kept in three-ring binders. By mistake, the printer who supplies us with our stationary sent a shipment of note papers without holes. This turned into a project for one gentleman who hadn't cared for any of the other activities offered. Over a period of several weeks, he punched holes in all the sheets we would need for months!

Stapling papers, folding newsletters, and stuffing envelopes are all jobs that need to be done on a regular basis. They can be organized into an assembly line where each client does one task that he is comfortable with. The "esprit de corps" that such a project generates is an absolute delight.

Special Events and Outings

Every holiday offers an opportunity to celebrate and a small party with decorations, treats, sing-alongs, and a few invited guests is an enjoyable way to do so. Keeping these occasions short so as not to overstimulate or overtire the clients is important. Birthdays of clients and staff may be celebrated with a small cake, prepared in secret by several clients and staff members, and a rousing chorus of "Happy Birthday."

Outings to local points of interest are a valuable part of a program during fine weather. It is best to avoid crowded places. Some enjoyable outings are picnics to a local park, a trip to the sugar bush for sugaring off with pancakes and syrup, a river cruise, a bus trip to view the autumn colors, and trips to local museums. Each client should be allowed to participate at his own level. Some clients can take in all the details and activity around them, while others are happy just to sit in the sun and chat. In every case, it is essential that each client feels safe with the group when being brought to an unfamiliar place and is assured that his individual needs will be met.

Films, which would seem a natural part of the program, have not proved to be successful. The dimming of the lights reduces sensory cues about the environment and causes some clients to become anxious or to turn inward. Poor visual perception and limited attention spans make films and slide presentations difficult for many clients to follow. One of the first indications of difficulty reported by many family members is that the client has lost interest in television. This should give us a clue.

Demonstrations of make-up, fashions, and flower arranging by local merchants are interesting. The interest is heightened, however, if clients are included, and especially if the demonstration involves familiar people, such as staff members, being made-up or modeling outlandish fashions.

The activities outlined above (and listed below) are but a sample to demonstrate selection and presentation. Ideas are always evolving, and the challenge lies in developing program ideas that meet the individual and group needs of the clients. The sensory components and socialization potential of all activities should be exploited.

List of Activities

GROSS MOTOR ACTIVITIES

Exercise

Walking

Dancing

Floor games: beanbag toss, shuffleboard, bowling, horseshoes, etc.

SELF-CARE ACTIVITIES

Dressing

Denture care

Mobility and transfers

Grooming, combing hair, skin care, manicure, make-up

Toileting

Meals and snacks

SOCIAL ACTIVITIES

Storytelling

Coffee klatch

Table games

Bingo

Sing-along

Orientation and wind-down

Parties

HOUSEKEEPING

Dusting

Mopping and sweeping

Washing and drying dishes

Tidying, sorting

Watering plants

Cleaning fishtank

MEAL PREPARATION

Sauces, soups, stews, casseroles

Steamed vegetables

Salads

Puddings

Pies and tarts

Muffins

Biscuits

Jams

Sandwiches

Table setting and clearing

Serving

CRAFTS

Bookmarks	Wood bits
Cutting boards	Christmas tree decorations
Hi-Q games	Harvest wreaths
Pompom animals	Cloth flowers
Decoupage plaques	Hasty notes

WORK-ORIENTED PROJECTS

Stuffing envelopes	Stapling and collating
Punching holes in paper	papers
	Stamping mail

SPECIAL EVENTS

Demonstrations	Outings

SENSORY ACTIVITIES

Perfumes	Music
Make-up	Picture books
Animals	Art
Rocking chair	Food tasting, finger foods
Massage	

7   The Presentation of Activities

Making Things Work

Once the appropriate activity has been identified and the level at which the client can participate has been determined, the key to successful completion lies in the way the activity is organized and how the client is initiated into and guided through it.

Organizing the Activity

Before an activity is set up for any client, it is important that the staff and volunteers be aware of its objectives, that is, the benefit that the client is expected to derive from participating in it. These objectives will determine how the activity is presented to the client and which steps will be highlighted as she is guided through it. For example, making Valentine's Day cards is intended to reinforce feelings of affection toward a loved one, recollect romantic and/or happy moments from the past, and help clients express their feelings for that person. In response to these objectives, the activity should include a discussion surrounding old photographs of the clients and their loved ones. An important part of the activity would be helping clients compose a note that expresses their feelings for their loved one. If the activity is limited to the actual making of the card, it would fall short of its objectives.

The next aspect of organization involves breaking the activity down into its individual steps and arranging them into a logical sequence. This must be done in detail, since many activities involve a number of steps which the normal person takes for granted and which may stymie the person with planning and sequencing problems. Each step is then reviewed in terms of the materials and equipment required, the type of instructions the client will be able to follow, and the visual and tactile reinforcers that may be used to trigger a habitual or overlearned pattern on the part of the client. The sensory experiences that can be drawn to the client's attention are also identified, and the client's ability to perform each step is determined. Steps that are too difficult for the client, such as measuring ingredients, should be done by the staff beforehand.

A distraction-free location appropriate for the activity is then chosen. Before the client is brought to the area, all materials and equipment should be close at hand, but only those that are to be used for each particular step should be within the immediate sight or reach of the client. This will ensure that there will be no interruptions and that the activity will flow smoothly.

Initiating the Activity

Many clients find it difficult to get started on a task. Asked if they want to do something, they frequently answer "No". This perceived negativism is usually a response to the stress resulting from an inability to conceptualize what is expected, a difficulty in initiating, and the fear of failure. Program staff and caregivers can usually avoid this initial refusal by giving a clear directive rather than offering an option, by stating, "Let's go do the dishes," rather than "Would you like to do the dishes?" and by accompanying the directive with a concrete visual or tactile clue whenever possible. Inertia can often be overcome by giving the client specific instructions with regard to the first step, such as "Hold this" or "Stand up. Come with me," and continuing with these instructions until the client takes over independently. The helper must, however, remain in close touch with the client's reactions and be sensitive to genuine refusal or resistance.

Most familiar activities can be started this way for clients who have difficulty initiating or who habitually refuse. For example, encouraging this type of client to use the washroom is often difficult. In most cases, it is best to state simply, "It's time to go to the washroom." The client still has the option to refuse if she really does not need to go. If, however, her judgment is known to be questionable, further encouragement may take the form of "You'd better go before getting on the bus." Continued refusal can be handled by avoiding mention of the objective and just starting the client on the first step of the task, saying "Get up. Come this way" and leading her to the washroom. The familiar place may trigger a familiar pattern of behavior, and the client will usually follow through. If she continues to protest at this point, it is usually best to let the matter drop. If there is no protest, but the client still has not taken any initiative, the helper can go on to the next step, saying "Pull down your pants," and positioning her hands so that she can carry on. Unless the client is totally dependent, she will usually pick up the task somewhere along the line. Other examples would be: leading the client to the sink and placing her hands into the soapy water to start her washing dishes, or placing the fork in her hand to help her start eating. In most cases, the client has just forgotten the first steps. Once she is started, the automatic pattern takes over.

If the activity is new to the client, such as a craft, more care must be taken to overcome her fear of the unknown. Show the client an example of the finished product and explain briefly how it is made. Don't present an option about participating at this early stage unless the client voices a serious objection. Explain briefly and in simple terms the product's use and why she is going to make it:

"A toy for your grandson" or "To sell at the bazaar." Making the purpose of the activity clear is important, as it establishes motivation. If she forgets and should ask again "Why?" repeat your answer, using exactly the same simple words each time. Altering the wording may confuse her.

Once the purpose of the activity is clear to the client, show her each component part and demonstrate simply how the activity is done. Do not expect her to remember the process at this time, and make it clear that you will repeat the explanation as often as necessary. This will ease her anxiety about the new task and may dissipate some of her resistance. Draw her attention to any sensory experiences, such as smell or texture, which are associated with the activity. Take your time. An eager client who understands the task will likely make a move to start when she is ready, but a client who is reticent may be turned off if you try to rush her into the activity.

If the client remains hesitant about the activity, begin it yourself. Keep her attention on what you are doing by providing a simple commentary and reinforcing the purpose of the activity. Remember, attending to an activity is a bona fide level of involvement and the first step to active participation. You can push for further participation by asking the client to help you in the task by holding something or handing you something. In this way the activity is graded for the client and she is led into more and more involvement. She may eventually continue with the task herself.

A client who continues to resist at this point is probably having some other problem. She may not feel well or may need to go to the bathroom, or she may simply object to the activity. In any case, you have chosen the wrong activity or the wrong time, and it is best to drop the issue, attend to the client's problem, try something else, or allow a little time out.

Guiding Clients through an Activity

Once the activity is under way, its successful outcome depends largely on the quality of the guidance the client is given. Even if you have planned the activity well, be prepared to guide the client through steps that you may not have anticipated. For example, a client who has something in her hand and is directed to pick up another object may need to be reminded to put down the first object.

An accurate assessment of the client's perceptual, motor, and cognitive abilities is important here. It will help you anticipate how much help the client will need. A cardinal rule is: give only as much help as is absolutely necessary. Let the client take as much initiative as she can. Trying to guide her too closely may squelch her initiative or interfere with her planned course of action. Learn to stand back and watch what she does. Be prepared to help if she is heading for trouble, but don't interfere unnecessarily.

Guidance can be given with verbal, visual, and manual cues. Manual or "hand-over-hand" direction refers to touching or moving the client's body in the desired direction.

Verbal cues should be kept simple, with a minimum of substantives and explanations. They are most effective when reinforced with visual cues. If instructions must be repeated, the same words should be used each time, using a calm, rhythmic intonation. This helps to reinforce learning and establish a pattern, and it taps into one of the AD client's characteristically retained perceptions, that of rhythm. A quiet, subdued tone of voice will minimize distraction and anxiety on the client's part. Instructions should be faded out as soon as it is obvious that the client knows what she is doing.

Manual direction, that is, touch, can be helpful when it is combined with verbal and visual cues. It is important to keep the touch within the client's line of sight, since an unexpected touch may be disconcerting to her. If you are going to guide a person's movement outside her line of sight, warn her first. Never attempt to move a client's body by force. Pushing and pulling will elicit either resistance or total passivity. Neither is desirable. The intention is to guide and encourage the client's muscles to make the effort in the right direction. Gentle pressure, light taps, or a firm touch over the muscle group to be used will usually facili-

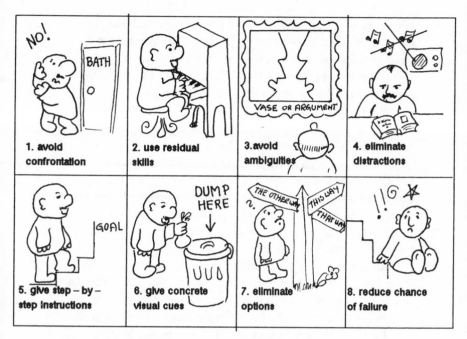

Eight axioms of management. (1) Rather than attempting to inform the client of the truth when he or she seems to be mistaken, try to see things from his or her perspective. (2) Keep the client actively using whatever skills he or she has retained. (3) Make sure that all sensory input to the client can be interpreted in only one way—the right way. (4) Keep extraneous stimuli, such as background noise, to a minimum. (5) Separate each task into its individual steps and give one instruction at a time. Keep to the logical sequence of the task. (6) Support verbal instructions with visual cues, such as the actual object being discussed or a demonstration of the movement required. (7) Avoid asking the client to make a choice unless the options are obvious to him or her and are presented in concrete terms. (8) Identify potential sources of difficulty and eliminate as many as possible before inviting the client to participate in an activity.

tate active movement on the client's part. Once a client is comfortable being touched, verbal cues can be faded out and the activity can be guided with unobtrusive manual cues alone. This minimizes the distraction and imparts more of a sense of independence on the part of the client. Make sure that the client really needs the guidance you are giving, and fade out all assistance as soon as possible.

Coping with Problems or Failure

When a client is having difficulty in any task, try to discern the source of her difficulty before offering a solution. An example comes to mind here. A gentleman was offered a sandwich from a tray brimming with lovely sandwiches. Although he had said that he would like one, when the tray was presented, his face dropped. He stared at the tray and finally declined. A staff member took one sandwich off the tray and offered it to him individually. He brightened up, accepted it happily, and ate it with relish. What had happened? The gentleman was not refusing the sandwich because he did not want it. He was unable to separate visually one sandwich from the pile on the tray, and so he could not select one. Rather than risk embarrassment, he withdrew. Encouraging him to eat would only have increased his discomfort. The staff member who took the time to identify the source of his difficulty was able to offer an unobtrusive and effective solution.

Sometimes a client's approach to a task may seem inappropriate. It is important to think before interjecting. Is her way of doing it really unacceptable, or are you imposing your own standards? She can eat her mashed potatoes with a spoon. Interrupting her and trying to give her a fork instead may confuse and disconcert her. On the other hand, a fork will not do for eating soup. In this case, it is best not to draw her attention to the error, but to substitute the spoon as unobtrusively as possible. The error was yours for having left the fork on the table in the first place.

There may be times when a client continues to have problems with a task and your assistance seems to be getting her deeper into difficulties. It is best to stop, pull back from the task, and approach it again. There may be something you overlooked in the initial set-up. For example, a

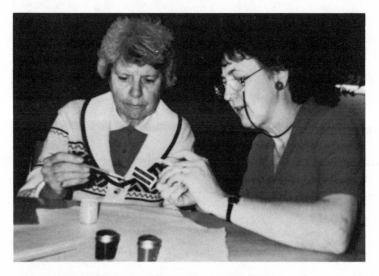

A helping hand must continue to involve the client.

lady was to chop celery for a stew. The staff member placed the knife in her right hand and the celery in her left and gave her instructions to chop. The lady did nothing, despite the fact that the task was well within her ability. The staff member guided her hands in the cutting motion. The client was passive and kept her eyes closed. On further encouragement, she made several faint and unsuccessful efforts to perform. Something was wrong, but she could not express the problem. With a flash of insight, the staff member removed the knife and the celery and presented it again, this time placing both items on the cutting board and repeating the instructions. The lady opened her eyes, took the knife in her left hand, and the celery in her right, and proceeded to chop the celery up quite nicely.

Many activities consist of several steps that are too difficult for the clients. These are usually done by staff members beforehand. However, if a difficult step occurs in midcourse of an activity, the temptation is to remove the activity and do it for the client. This may rob her of her sense of independence and accomplishment. Whenever possible, keep the client involved during the process while you offer more help or guidance. "Let me help you with that" is a more appropriate approach than "Let me do that for you."

Despite all efforts to minimize chances of failure and to preserve the client's self-esteem and sense of accomplishment, mistakes are made and projects do "bomb." The key is to reduce the negative impact of such an experience on the client. If you are not sure about the outcome of a particular project, make it clear to the client from the start. Let her know that you are both embarking on an experiment, and assure her that its failure will be no reflection on her.

Providing Positive Reinforcement

Positive reinforcement, given on a regular basis throughout the activity, will let the client know that she is on the right track. A simple nod or reassuring glance may be all that is needed. Be careful, though, not to distract the client just to let her know that she is doing fine.

When an activity is successfully completed and you and the client have expended considerable effort toward this achievement, positive feelings need an outlet. It is important to resist the temptation to "overpraise" the client. One lady became quite disconcerted when she was praised for having set the table. Although it had taken considerable effort, it was a simple and familiar task to her. A simple "Thank you" would probably have made her feel better. Most of the activities selected for a program are easy, and clients, for the most part, are aware of that. Their pleasure is in finding things that they can do. The gratification comes mainly from participating in the activity and gaining a sense of being able to contribute. This is not to say that effort should not be praised, only that it should be acknowledged realistically. A former nuclear physicist in the program once said, "I may be demented, but I am not stupid."

The techniques outlined in this chapter are aimed at facilitating meaningful activity by the clients in a way that will preserve their dignity and take full advantage of their remaining abilities.

8 Clients' Reactions to the Program

The Realities

It would be wonderful if every client were eager to attend the program and enjoyed it thoroughly from the start. However, there are always a number of clients who find it difficult to adjust. They may be reluctant to accept the idea of being involved in the program. They may resist leaving the security of home or find it difficult to stay in an unfamiliar setting for a whole day. These problems may persist for several months, since poor memory, limited insight, conceptual difficulties, and visuospatial and temporal distortions all interfere with the client's ability to adjust to change. If the program is to be of benefit to either, both client and caregiver need to receive much support during this potentially stressful period.

Introducing the Program

The client's first encounter with program staff and the idea of attending a day program should ideally occur at his own home, where he can meet the staff member, who will remain a consistent contact for him and his family, under relaxed and familiar circumstances. The staff member is also better able to evaluate the client's suitability for the program if the client is relaxed and comfortable. The decision to accept or not to accept a client into the program should be based mainly on the client's potential to benefit from social contacts and meaningful activity, and on the family's need for respite.

Even the most suitable clients often respond negatively to the first suggestion of attending the program. The idea threatens to confront them with problems they may have been denying and raises all the fears and anxieties associated with the unknown. Some clients fear that this interview is the beginning of placement procedures. At this time the staff member can model a supportive and positive attitude for the family. He may acknowledge the client's fears and apprehension and assure him that he will be afforded all the support he needs in this new venture. In a positive vein, the staff member points out the benefits for the client of attending a day program. At no time is the client forced to make any commitment or made to feel pressured into attending. Usually, the program experience is offered on a trial, "Come out and see what it is all about" basis.

The client may, in an effort to be polite, agree to attend the program, but, once the staff member has left, the client may voice some very negative feelings to the family. Family members are warned of this possibility and are advised to acknowledge the client's feelings, substantiate his anxiety, and offer him emotional support. If family members understand the basis for the client's negative feelings, they can give this support and avoid confrontation. They can maintain a positive attitude and refrain from making an issue of the client's resistance.

Helping Clients Leave Home

Leaving home to attend the program for the first time is often stressful. Even the client who seemed enthusiastic about having a chance to meet new friends and have a good time may become ambivalent or even resistant when it is time to leave home. A staff member should be on the van every time it arrives to collect the client. This provides an added measure of security. If it is anticipated that the client may find the first morning particularly difficult, arrangements should be made for the staff member who made the initial contact to be on the van for that first trip.

Every effort is made to help the client adjust to the new routine with as little stress as possible. Family members may accompany the client on his first visit to the program. New clients may be eased into the program by coming for only a short period on the first day; in this way, they are reassured that they will be returning home.

The fear of venturing out may subside after only a few visits, or it may persist for a long time. Sometimes it even becomes a pattern. The staff member is met each morning with a recital from the client of reasons he is unable to come. The staff member's approach to helping the client come out may vary from calm reassurance to firm direction, depending on the client's needs, but the approach must always be sensitive to the client's level of anxiety or resistance. One gentleman in "Day Away" was so stressed by going out that efforts to include him in the program had to be abandoned. He would start out toward the van and back off at the last minute. His fear of leaving home verged on panic and could not be overcome by any amount of reassurance. One lady, who had been coming to the program regularly, came to the door one morning and stated that she no longer wanted to attend the program. Her sister had started taking her out shopping once weekly, and this outing was sufficient for her. Her wishes had to be respected.

Sometimes the process of coming to the program must be broken down into small steps that are taken one at a time. One lady absolutely refused to come. Both the family and the staff agreed that the program would be very beneficial to her if only she could overcome her fear of venturing out. A staff member visited her at home and took her out for a walk, then encouraged her to sit in the car, ride around the block, and eventually, drive down to the program. This procedure was repeated three times before she was able to board the van on her own. Although she had enjoyed her experience at the program, that fear of venturing out welled up each morning when it came time to leave home. It became a pattern that the family learned to accept and deal with.

Because clients generally attend the program only once weekly, it is essential that consistency be maintained. The program day must be structured into a fairly rigid pattern. This helps clients adjust to the routine more readily. It is helpful if the routine at home in preparation for departure is consistent, as well. Families are encouraged to establish such a routine, and to use the same words and expressions whenever they talk about the program.

Clients who are used to sleeping late in the morning, or who have a hard time dressing and grooming, find the early pick-up difficult. Their families are sometimes so stressed by the rush that the program becomes counterproductive. If the client can be driven to the program later in the day, accommodations for late arrival should be arranged.

Dealing with Clients' Negative Reactions

Although the program day is structured to accommodate clients' cognitive deficits and to provide a secure and predictable environment, a number of clients will continue to experience episodes of anxiety or distress. These problems are often the result of memory loss. The client does not remember how he will get home or whether a loved one is waiting for him somewhere. During these times, frequent reassurances from staff are helpful. If the client can be distracted from his anxiety and become involved in an interesting task, the agitation usually subsides.

Unfortunately, some clients do not relate positively to any activities offered in the program and therefore cannot be relieved of their anxiety. These are often former businessmen or executives who previously engaged in little social or leisure activity outside their work. They are also people who premorbidly were asocial, demanding, and very independent. Day programs are not usually suitable for these clients, as they find it difficult to function well in a group setting, tend to have particular problems adjusting to a state of relative dependence, and do not respond well to leisure activities. "Day Away"'s ability to accommodate these clients in a positive way has, thus far, been limited. Families of these clients are encouraged to seek psychiatric support, directive and supportive counseling, and in-home respite and activation services. The Home Assistance Program offers assistance in these cases.

If recurring periods of agitation are documented, a pattern usually emerges. In many cases, these episodes occur at the same time each day and can be related to some regular event in the client's former schedule. Women often become restless at about midafternoon, the time when their children used to come home from school and they started to prepare dinner. A particularly involving activity, one that approximates the task the client used to do at that time of day, can be planned at that time for the client who exhibits this difficulty.

Some clients simply need a "time-out" at some point in the day. One lady in "Day Away" regularly slipped into the cloakroom and looked at her coat and hat for a while, apparently needing to touch base with something familiar. Permitted this time alone, she would come back to the program calmer and ready to resume her activity.

Some clients become so distressed that they desperately want to leave the program. These are usually clients in whom the disease has progressed far and who are experiencing hallucinations or episodes of paranoia. Staff members must be prepared to deal with such clients to ensure their safety, their caregiver's peace of mind, and the comfort of other clients in the program. Ideally, staff members will be able to see an episode building and take measures to distract or reassure the client before it becomes a crisis. Once the client is in a crisis, he needs very special handling. He needs someone to be on his side and confirm his feelings of anxiety. Efforts to restrain him physically and arguments will only create an adversary situation between the client and the staff member and increase the client's agitation and resentment. It often helps to permit the client to leave the premises under the unobtrusive supervision of a staff member. Another staff member leaves the room by a different exit, comes around to intercept the client, approaching him from the front, greets him in a friendly manner, takes him by the arm, and leads him out for a walk. By the time they return to the program, the client's agitation has subsided and he is able to resume his activity. In extreme cases, two staff members will have to alternate several times. As one becomes the "restraining foe," the other takes over as the "rescuing friend."

It is unrealistic to sustain such a situation for an extended period of time, especially because it causes the client so much distress. Clients in whom such behavior persists are usually referred for psychiatric intervention. In many cases, however, the clients are reassured that their efforts to leave will not result in negative reactions from the staff, and these episodes stop. One gentleman in "Day Away" continued to have difficulty for about three months. Eventually, however, he was able to reassure himself when he felt the anxiety welling up by saying to the staff, "It's O.K. It's not you. It's only my problem. I'm just feeling crazy again."

Providing Support for Caregivers

Although every effort is made to accommodate the client, the caregiver also needs support. The husband who has witnessed his wife's stress on leaving home but who does not see her later, enjoying herself at the program, may find that the morning's experience overshadows his whole day. Whereas most clients quickly forget the stress of leaving home once they become involved in the activities and social groups, their caregivers may continue to stew about it. Rather than enjoying their day of respite, they worry about how their loved ones are doing and feel guilty for having subjected them to that stress.

It happens occasionally that a client who seemed to have

had a pleasant day in the program comes home and complains bitterly to his family. These complaints are usually the result of fatigue related to anxiety about being in an unfamiliar place, and they eventually subside. Because he is unable to pinpoint the specific cause for his distress, the client tends to paint a black picture of the whole experience. This is very disconcerting to the caregiver, who takes the complaints at face value, and it may result in the client's being withdrawn from the program prematurely. Caregivers must be advised that these complaints are quite common. Further reassurance may be derived from regular meetings between the staff and the caregiver. The caregiver may also be given the opportunity to come in and view the program through the one-way mirror.

The journal that travels with the client to and from the program may serve as another valuable source of information about the client's activities during the day. Family support groups provide mutual help and a chance to share feelings. If the program is to work successfully for the client, the caregiver must be supported in maintaining a positive outlook through what may be some difficult times.

A Case History

The following case history portrays my work with one family and the efforts that went into bringing Mrs. Mary A. to "Day Away." It demonstrates how much support both a client and his family may need to make the experience a success. It also illustrates a number of important points: (1) if the proper groundwork is laid, serious behavior problems can be avoided; (2) resistance and negativism are expressions of the client's feelings and must be addressed sympathetically; and (3) if behavior is to change, the feelings that spawned it must be changed first.

Mrs. A.'s referral to "Day Away" came from her family doctor, who had made a diagnosis of Alzheimer's disease on the basis of a CAT scan, an E.E.G., and neuropsychological testing. She is sixty-five years old, a housewife, and in good physical health. She has three adult children by a previous marriage. One son and one daughter live with their own families in town. One daughter lives quite a distance away. Mrs. A. has a sister overseas who is severely disabled with Alzheimer's disease.

Mrs. A.'s husband, who is seven years her junior, works full time in a local factory. He has had two heart attacks and suffers from Crohn's disease and arthritis. These chronic ailments limit his tolerance for emotional stress.

Over a period of three years, Mr. A. had noticed a gradual decline in his wife's ability to cope with the household. She frequently left the stove on. Her normally fastidious grooming had deteriorated. Her memory for recent happenings had become markedly impaired. She was spending large sums of money on foolish things. Mr. A. suspected that she had removed some items from stores without paying for them. She had become short-tempered and subject to catastrophic reactions. Mr. A. often came home from work to find that some treasured object had been thrown out or destroyed or that Mrs. A. had sustained some inexplicable cuts or burns. Whenever she was asked about these things, Mrs. A. would become defensive, and a heated argument would develop. Mrs. A. frequently hid or misplaced objects and later accused others of having taken them. She became unable to carry on any but the most superficial of conversations.

By the time Mr. A. sought medical help, he had completely taken over the management of the household and was going to work each day worried about what he would find on his return. He was coping with the numerous disruptions that resulted from his wife's misdoings. In addition, he was suffering the emotional loss of his companion and helpmate. As a result of his wife's inability to plan entertainment, her poor tolerance of large groups, and his own reluctance to leave her alone during the evenings, Mr. A. had become socially isolated.

Because Mrs. A. had maintained her impeccable social skills throughout this time, friends and even family members who came into the home for short visits had no indication that there was anything seriously wrong. They suggested that Mr. A.'s complaints were exaggerations, based more on dissatisfaction with the marriage than on any real problem. Consequently, Mr. A. was unable to share his burden with any of his friends or his family.

When I first contacted Mr. A. about the referral, he was very apprehensive. No one had told Mrs. A. about the nature of her problem. He had no idea how to approach it with her. Mrs. A.'s children did not want their mother to be upset and did not believe that outside help was warranted.

I arranged to meet with Mr. A. in a restaurant near his home. Much of the time was spent in Mr. A.'s expressing his feelings about the situation, telling of the incredible things that Mary had done lately, and just feeling relieved that someone finally knew what he was talking about. This type of venting is important. Before they have contact with someone who understands, family members feel totally isolated with their problem. Many of the things that happen at home are just too incredible to share with the uninitiated. Imagine facing a supper served up on dishes that had been washed in lemon oil instead of detergent, or coming home to a wife who has taken a whole package of laxatives.

During the course of this meeting, it became apparent that Mr. A. knew very little about Alzheimer's disease. I explained the physical background of the disease and helped Mr. A. relate his wife's behavior to specific aspects of her illness. Mr. A. was relieved to learn that these behaviors were not a reflection of her feelings toward him but, rather, manifestations of a disease process. Mr. A. acknowledged that his stepchildren needed to have this information, too, so that they could understand what was happening to their mother.

We then established that Mrs. A. had to be told of her problem. There were two basic reasons for this. First, there had to be good reason for a stranger to come to her home, ask her questions, and invite her to come to a day program. Giving a fictitious reason would only create a web of untruths that would eventually collapse, destroying Mrs. A.'s faith in everyone concerned. Second, Mrs. A. was probably already aware that something was seriously wrong. Her short temper and irritability were at least partly the result of her efforts at covering up. If she was told that her difficulties were due to an illness and were not her fault, she would eventually find it easier to cope and to accept help. I explained that she needed to know that others were aware of her problem, were willing to help her, and thought no less of her because of her illness.

Mr. A. was concerned about mentioning Alzheimer's disease to his wife. She was aware of her sister's condition and would be distraught at facing the same fate. We agreed to call it a "memory loss" for the time being. But I cautioned Mr. A. against denying to Mrs. A. that she had the disease. She would encounter the word eventually during her involvement in the program. Other clients talk about Alzheimer's, and the word is on a sign on the door to the program area, so Mrs. A.'s diagnosis could not be hidden from her indefinitely. I stressed the importance of being gentle but honest. We agreed that a family meeting would help to get all of these issues into the open and would be the best solution.

The family meeting started off as a tense situation, everyone sitting in the family room, going through the social pleasantries, and waiting for me to tell Mary the real reason for my visit. I told her that I work with people who have memory problems and that I had come to see her because I understood that she, too, has been having problems with her memory. Mary made no objections to these statements. In fact, she was quite eager to talk about it. She admitted that such problems are very upsetting and that she was often quite frightened by what was happening.

Had I asked her, point blank, if she was having problems with her memory, she would probably have answered "No." She may even have become irate. Most likely she would have insisted that she does all the housework, that her husband helps occasionally, but that she can do everything without difficulty. The situation may have deteriorated into an argument, with Mr. A. recalling numerous episodes of memory loss and Mary becoming defensive.

She needed the structure of several preparatory statements such as:

"I work in a program that helps people with memory problems."

"Memory problems are really quite common."

"They can be very upsetting and make you become angry or frustrated, especially when people ask you questions that you can't answer or tell you that you've done things that you cannot remember."

"I understand that you have been having problems with your memory lately. Have any of these things happened to you?"

Mary was able to process this information. She did not feel threatened and was able to admit that she did have some difficulty. It was then easy to lead her through some recent happenings and illustrate her need for help.

Had she denied memory problems, I would not have tried to convince her. Instead, I would have explored other identifiable problems such as "nerves," depression, headaches, etc., until we hit upon something to which she could relate. Few persons with AD will, unless they are confronted, insist that they are absolutely fine. They do not feel well and usually just need to be given a structure within which they can describe their problems.

The key in such an initial encounter is to explore various avenues of approach gently and sensitively, remembering that establishing the client's trust is the primary objective. At the first indication of resistance or defensiveness from the client, the worker is advised to back off and try another approach. It is important to remember that we are dealing with a person who has limited insight and limited ability to abstract, along with a very strong need to maintain control. Attempts to argue a point will only alienate that person.

In cases where no common ground can be found, it is best for the worker just to visit socially, promise to return another time, and part with the client on good terms. Several visits may be necessary before the client is comfortable enough to lower his guard and admit to having a problem. During the year and a half that I worked at the program, I encountered only one client with whom this approach did not eventually lead to a workable relationship. In this gentleman the disease was very far advanced, and he had psychiatric problems of long standing.

Mary responded well to this first meeting. She was apprehensive about the suggestion of a day program but was assured that no one would force her into anything. I invited her to come out one day and just look around. She agreed to this offer.

As part of the intake assessment, I administered the Hierarchic Dementia Scale. I remained vigilant to Mary's reaction and was prepared to stop whenever I sensed that it was causing her excessive anxiety. She had some questions about it and complained that the tasks, such as the block puzzle, were childish. I agreed that some of the items seemed silly, but that they would help me find out which tasks she could perform with ease and what kind of things were difficult for her. I explained that, when someone has a memory problem such as hers, other functions, such as the ability to organize things or plan jobs, may also be impaired. These exercises, I said (it is best to avoid the word *test*), would help me identify the kind of help she could best benefit from. Mary's recent memory was so poor that this explanation had to be repeated frequently throughout the session.

Some test items may confront the client with a blatant deficit, which can be very upsetting and must be presented with care. In this case, Mary was unable to write her own name. She persisted in trying and became more and more upset with her inability. Efforts on my part to pass it over by saying "That's O.K." and move on to another item would have upset her further. It was not O.K. Mary was devastated by the fact that, as an adult, she could not write her own name. She needed someone to validate her feelings and give her emotional support. I agreed with her that it was a bad situation and coached her through the laborious process, which finally resulted in a deformed but legible signature.

Mary's poor memory proved to be the saving grace in this situation. After a few tears and some hand holding, she forgot the upset and was ready to continue with the assessment. Her family, who had witnessed this episode, did not recover so quickly. Therefore, after explaining briefly to Mary what the assessment had told me, I left her in the parlor with her daughter and met with the rest of the family in the kitchen. We went through each test item they had observed. I interpreted Mary's responses in terms of her disability and related each response to practical situations.

If the family can cope with seeing the client's deficits graphically exposed, it is useful to administer this assessment in their presence. It helps them realize the extent of the client's disability and readjust their expectations to more realistic levels. A family who has been exposed to such a demonstration needs explanations and support, however.

Sometimes this interpretation can be done in the presence of the client. Many families are afraid to confront the client with such a situation but feel guilty about doing things behind the client's back. Clients who are aware that something that concerns them is being discussed may become quite upset and accuse their families of plotting against them. Presenting the information in the presence of the client and in a manner that everyone can understand may avoid this cycle of guilt and paranoia. It is a matter that requires the worker's careful consideration. In this case I gave Mary the basic information, but when the family requested a more detailed explanation that would have been beyond Mary's ability to understand, I chose to exclude her from the second discussion.

Following my discussion with the family, I returned to the parlor and invited Mary into the kitchen to help me prepare a cup of tea. I often use this fairly complex task to evaluate the client's ability to plan, sequence, and follow through with an activity. Mary had a great deal of difficulty initiating. Once started, she tended to perseverate in placing cups on the tray and would have emptied the cupboard had I not suggested that five cups would be enough. As long as she was able to follow an automatic pattern of behaviors, she could perform satisfactorily, but when she was distracted by conversation, she had much difficulty returning to the task.

These observations, along with the history and the results of Mary's H.D.S., indicated that she was suffering from a serious handicap and must have been working very hard to maintain even her currently limited level of function. The assessment also underscored the fact that she was not safe at home alone for any extended period of time and that her husband's worries were well founded.

This first meeting with Mary and her family seemed to have gone very smoothly. Mr. A. was told about the family support groups and was encouraged to attend. He was still very concerned about the future for himself and for Mary. I told him that plans would include a referral to the Regional Health Unit's Home Care program to provide some home support, as well as contact with Regional Special Services to help him sort out his financial situation and determine how he could obtain companion service for Mary while he was at work. Mary had agreed to try "Day Away." The children had gained some insight into the problems that their mother and stepfather were experiencing.

Before leaving, I warned the family that Mary might, in retrospect, react negatively to the visit and later resist going to the program. I suggested that it would take some time for her to accept the program and the home help but that we would all work together to help her adjust.

The next morning, this prediction came true. A very distressed Mr. A. phoned the program. Mary had become very upset when I left. She had been agitated all night, asking him repeatedly if she had the same disease that had incapacitated her sister. She insisted that she would do away with herself if she did. She would have no part of "Day

Away" and refused to have anyone come into the house as a companion or homemaker. She accused him of not loving her anymore. Mr. A. was afraid to go to work and leave her in this state.

I sympathized with his problems and explained that such a reaction was not uncommon. Mary had been confronted with many new ideas and impending changes. She was frightened by all this and did not have the resources to deal with her fear rationally.

I asked him if she could be joked out of her despairing mood and suicidal thoughts. He said yes, that she could. He had told her not to do it just now because he hadn't picked out a good cemetery plot yet. The fact that this somewhat macabre humor could make her laugh suggested that Mary's thoughts of suicide were not serious, even though they were very distressing for Mr. A. It was her way of saying that she was frightened and did not know what to do. I encouraged him to be supportive, to hear her out, and to maintain a positive attitude about the plans despite her objections. If she persisted in this type of talk, I suggested that he distract her with a change of topic.

It soon became obvious that Mr. A. was too upset himself to follow through with these suggestions. I asked him to put Mary on the telephone while he listened in on the extension, and I modeled some of these supportive techniques for him. I told Mary that I understood how upsetting all these new things were. The prospects of going to a new place and having strangers in her home were all frightening, but Mr. A., her children, and I would all help her. In response to her questions about AD, I told her that memory loss could be caused by any number of conditions and that right now we were concerned about helping her cope with it. After hearing these points repeated several times, Mary seemed to be placated. When she hung up the receiver, I suggested to Mr. A. that he ask a neighbor to come over and stay with Mary while he went to work. I would be over shortly to talk with Mary. He agreed and went to work.

That morning, Mary and I made tea and talked for about

two hours. In response to her questions about "Day Away," I explained that all the people who attended had memory problems. With regard to the homemaker companion, I explained that no one would come in to take over her home. The lady who would come would help her do the things that she used to like doing before this problem started. Mary frequently interjected, saying that she could cope on her own. I reflected to her that she could do many things but that she had difficulty starting and organizing jobs. If someone helped her get organized, she would be able to do things like baking, housekeeping, and even some crafts that she had enjoyed in the past. Each time we went through this, Mary agreed. Then, out of the blue, she would say, "But I'm not going to the program" or "I won't have anyone in the house." Then I would go through the whole explanation again. Consistent repetition is often necessary before the client can come to terms with a new idea.

When Mr. A. called home shortly before lunchtime, I told him that Mary was fairly well settled, repeated the vocabulary I had used to explain the homemaker and the "Day Away" to Mary, and encouraged him to use the very same words when he spoke to her about it. Mary and I made lunch. I told her that I would come the next morning to pick her up and take her to see the program. I called the neighbor and asked her to stay with Mary until Mr. A. returned from work. As it happened, the neighbor was a friend of the family who agreed to sit with Mary regularly until a paid homemaker companion could be arranged.

The next morning I arrived at Mary's home to find her in bed and refusing to get up. I spent some time sitting with Mary and going through my explanation of the program. I then simply held out her robe and told her to put it on. She responded immediately to this simple command but still insisted that she was not going out to the program.

We sat over tea and, again, I reaffirmed how frightening all this must be but assured her that I would stay with her and would take her home as soon as she wanted to leave. She agreed just to go for a ride in the car.

After much reassurance and repetition of my explanations, Mary eventually agreed to visit "Day Away." Once there, she joined into the activities quite easily and seemed to enjoy herself for the whole day. I drove her home at the end of the day, reviewed the day's events with her, and left the journal for Mr. A. to read. Mary did not express any negative feelings and seemed quite pleased with the experience.

That evening, however, Mr. A. called again. Mary was insisting that she would not return to the program. She claimed that there were only old people there and had many stories of strange happenings. Mr. A., too, was doubtful if she should return, as, according to Mary's description, the group did not seem to be appropriate for her. Furthermore, Mrs. A.'s son had insisted that Mary should not be forced into doing anything that upset her so much and had made it clear to Mary that he was not in favor of her going to the program. Mr. A. did not want to be involved in a conflict with his stepson.

I encouraged Mr. A. to read the journal, which outlined all the pleasant things that Mary had experienced during the day, and to try to reinforce to Mary the positive aspects of the program. I dissuaded him from suggesting to Mary that she was not going again. In a phone call to Mary's son, I explained the importance of the day away for Mary and the freedom from worry that day would mean for Mr. A. and requested his support. He agreed reluctantly.

For the next two weeks I collected Mary in my car and took her to the program. Each time we went through the same routine of getting her out of bed, and each time her response in the program was positive. Mr. A. visited the program one day to assure himself that Mary's negative reports were founded only on her anxiety about leaving home. Mary introduced him enthusiastically to her new friends. This gave them something to talk about at home and provided him with concrete material with which to reinforce the positive aspects of the program whenever she started to protest about going.

Mr. A. started to attend family support meetings and heard about other clients who had had difficulty adjusting to the program in the initial weeks. The other group members supported him and encouraged him to persist with Mary. He was still having to cope with Mary's questions about AD, her threats of suicide, and her hostile reactions whenever he insisted that she go. We kept in touch through almost daily telephone calls. This contact was important if Mr. A. was to see this adjustment period through.

In the meanwhile, program staff observed Mary closely, to determine if there were any aspects of the program which may have been contributing to her negative recollections. They noted that, if Mary was not given absolutely specific instructions when asked to perform a task, her response could be very impulsive, and the results were frequently embarrassing.

A particularly illustrative event occurred during Mary's second week in the program. A volunteer asked Mary to put some crackers out on the cheese platter. Before the volunteer could provide more explicit directions, Mary opened the box and dumped its contents—broken crackers and crumbs—over the cheese platter. Several clients noticed the incident and expressed their displeasure. Anyone could imagine Mary's embarrassment. Although she would not remember the incident that evening, the memory of having had a negative experience would certainly have colored her general impression of the day.

Because Mary's social skills belied the extent of her cognitive impairment, a special note was made on her individual treatment plan and pointed out to new volunteers. This note indicated that explicit instructions were essential to ensure that such embarrassments did not recur.

Mary's most consistent complaint to Mr. A. about the program was of one lady who often fretted about her husband who was coming to get her. Everyone, including Mary, knew that this lady's husband had died some time ago. I explained to Mary that this lady was really expressing her need for reassurance and was worried because she couldn't remember how she was going to get home that afternoon. I suggested that Mary may be just the person to comfort this lady when she was so upset. Despite her cognitive disability, Mary could relate to this lady's anxiety and could see a role for herself in helping her. This lady's need became a major motivation for Mary to continue to attend the program. She was needed there.

When Mr. A. was first told of this, he thought that it was merely a ploy to encourage Mary's attendance. He was surprised to hear that Mary's role with other clients was, in fact, real. He acknowledged that Mary did have a talent for making people feel comfortable, and that she had always been a very empathetic person. But he had become so used to seeing Mary's deficits that he had lost sight of her very real assets. This change of perspective was a very positive step for him.

As Mary's resistance to the program diminished, we decided that she was ready to go on the van. The first morning, we received a desperate call from the staff member who was on van duty. Mary was still in bed. The neighbor could not get her up, and the van could not wait. I made another trip, got Mary up, and took her to the program.

That afternoon, however, she went home on the van without difficulty. From that time onward Mary rode to the program regularly without major incident. There were still regular evening calls from Mr. A. saying that Mary was not coming the next day. Each time, however, he was encouraged to be firm, and Mary did come.

Getting Mary to accept the homemaker was another matter. To introduce her to the idea of having someone helping her at home, I visited twice weekly for a period of two weeks. We cooked and cleaned together and enjoyed Mr. A.'s reaction to coming home to a prepared meal. We went for walks and stopped for coffee in a local coffeeshop.

On the third week, I told Mary that I would be bringing a colleague who would be doing similar things with her on a regular basis. In this way my relationship with Mary formed a bridge to introduce the homemaker companion. As we worked out the activity plan and activity routine together, Mary was reassured that the homemaker would continue doing all the same things we had enjoyed.

Once the first homemaker was established, we introduced a second one to provide more time and to expose Mary to two familiar people. In case one became sick or went on vacation, Mary would not be confronted with a stranger.

The entire process of introducing Mary to the program took a period of about four months. It required a lot of work, foresight, and patience. But, as a result, Mary was involved in a program, both at home and at "Day Away," which gave her an opportunity to be active and productive and to have regular contact with other people. A network of home supervision was set up that permitted Mr. A. to go to work with peace of mind. It also linked him into a system that could provide him with ongoing support.

Over the next months, Mr. A. became more friendly with other family support group members. They visited mutually and made reciprocal sitting arrangements for evenings. I helped Mr. A. fill out placement papers for the time when he would no longer be able to care for Mary at home. We kept in close touch so that Mr. A. would have someone to call on when things became difficult. This type of ongoing support for the family is essential to the maintenance of an AD client in the community. Because new situations keep arising, the client's condition deteriorates, sitters change, and caregivers just get tired, this type of support must be permanently installed. There is no time when one can say, "That's done, now things are fine."

We had an example of just such a case when Mary's day for attending the program was changed to include her in a more appropriate group. Her resistance surfaced again. The old system of supports had to be reenlisted. This time Mary's adjustment was quicker, but it would not have occurred had the support system not been available.

The techniques used in handling Mary and her resistance to the plans we had made may be viewed by some as manipulation of the individual. If a healthy person had been handled this way, it would have been just that. We are dealing, however, with a person whose ability to process and retain information and make rational judgments is severely impaired. We must, therefore, make some decisions for them. The decisions, however, must be based on an accurate evaluation of the situation. This evaluation must include an ongoing sensitivity to the client's emotional state, as well as judgments as to the origin of any negative emotions he expresses.

If Mary had reacted negatively to the program once she was there and had continued to do so after four or five visits, I would not have persisted in encouraging her to go. If she had been so resistant to leaving home that my efforts to get her out could not have been maintained on a good-natured level, I would not have persisted. These were ongoing judgments that were made and reevaluated at each step in the process. Mary's response and eventual capitulation each day indicated quite clearly that her initial resistance stemmed from fear of change and the unknown. This was what we had to help her overcome.

The issue of whether Mary believed that she had AD was never resolved. We continued to repeat the original explanation each time she brought it up. Eventually she would answer her own question, saying, "I have a memory loss." Her husband and I agreed that, since this seemed to satisfy her, there was nothing to be gained from pursuing accuracy.

9   Mobility

It is a frequent source of consternation to those who care for persons with AD that, despite the clients' apparent physical well-being, they often have much difficulty moving about. What would seem like a simple trip across a room becomes a major effort. Rising from a chair or sitting down on the toilet often presents problems. Getting in and out of a car may become a frustrating experience. Some of these difficulties may be alleviated for both clients and caregivers by the institution of helping techniques.

In order to move about successfully and safely, we depend on more than good muscles, bones, and joints. Balance and navigation also depend on good body image, motor planning, and spatial awareness. We must be able to assess the surrounding area, determine the distance of objects, and judge their spatial relation to each other and to ourselves. Then we must plan a clear route to the destination. We must be able to call on the right muscle groups to initiate movement in the desired direction. Once under way, we must keep a lookout for obstacles and judge whether our body will fit through a space.

These are all fairly complex maneuvers for the client who is spatially and posturally insecure. Therefore, we can understand why many clients are reluctant to move about independently or do so slowly and cautiously. Careful observation will reveal which areas are causing the movement-impaired client the most difficulty and should suggest some effective methods of intervention. The following techniques can be used to facilitate movement.

Walking

Although the client may show no signs of physical impairment, perceptual dysfunction can seriously impede her mobility.

- Walking through a crowded area is threatening for the client who is spatially insecure. It often helps if you offer her your arm and lead, rather than push, her through the area.
- A client may be able to move more securely if she is given a concrete visual target to head for, such as "the blue chair," and if the route to the destination is clear of obstacles.
- It may be necessary to break down a long trip into several "legs."
- Warning the client of obstacles and irregularities in the terrain may add to her security.
- A client who has an irregular gait or who has some physical impairment will walk more evenly if a rhythm is established. Take her arm firmly and use your body to set a somewhat exaggerated rhythm to the steps. This will encourage a more normal gait than verbal instructions alone would.
- A client who has difficulty coordinating the movement of a cane or a walker often responds well to instructions given in single words in the cadence of the walk, e.g., "Step, walker, step, walker."

Rising from a Chair

This can become a serious problem for the more severely motor-impaired client. It can be frustrating and time consuming for both client and staff. When the task is approached in a step-by-step fashion, some of this frustration can be alleviated.

- The first step in rising from a chair is to move forward in the seat. Therefore, before attempting to transfer a client from a chair, ensure that she is positioned well forward.
- The second step is to position the feet back slightly under the seat of the chair and flat on the ground. The heels may be raised slightly, especially if the client has tight heelcords.
- The next step for the client is to lean forward, bring her body weight out over the feet, and push off with her hands either from her knees or from the arms of the chair. It sometimes helps to give the client gentle but firm pressure on the nape of the neck (not the back of the head) to bring the head forward and bring her center of gravity over her feet just as she is making the effort to rise. Some clients find it easier to execute this maneuver on the count of three, so their efforts and the staff members' efforts can be coordinated.
- If the client does not succeed in rising from the chair and standing on the first try, you may offer her a hand to help her balance herself, but avoid trying to pull her up. It may confuse her in her efforts to rise, and you may be left supporting her whole weight. This is not safe for you or for the client. Rather, let her back down gently and try again.
- A client who is very weak or who has poor balance is likely to need a walker for ambulating. Position the walker in front of her and let her pull up on it while you guide her as she shifts her weight.

Seating a Client in a Chair or on the Toilet

This is sometimes as difficult as rising and can be facilitated with the following techniques.

- Point out the chair as you approach it with the client.
- Approach the chair from the front and direct the client to

bend slightly and place her hand on the chair arm on the opposite side.

- Then, while keeping her hand on the arm of the chair, direct her to "turn, turn, turn," taking small steps until she is positioned with her back square to the chair. You may guide her by putting firm pressure on her hip and nudging her in the right direction.
- Once she is positioned, direct her to reach back for the other arm of the chair and ease herself down.
- Some clients have difficulty flexing their hips at this point. A little downward pressure with your hand on the nape of her neck may help her get down.
- For severely motor-impaired clients, a commode chair with arms placed over the toilet is very helpful.

Some complex maneuvers, such as getting in and out of the car, become even more difficult if the client is given time to "think" about what she is to do. At this point she may realize that she cannot remember how to go about it and may get "stuck." It often helps to keep up a casual conversation as you approach the car with her, open the door, and gently and unobtrusively position her for entry into the vehicle. The long-established pattern of movement will often take over.

In all these techniques, the principle applies of providing only as much help as the client really needs. Too much help can be as confusing as too little.

Conclusion

Alzheimer's disease presents those who work in the area with a number of challenges. Most obvious and highly publicized among these has been the search for a cause and a cure. The first step in that direction was the recognition of deterioration in cognitive functions as a real disease entity. Another equally important challenge is the maintenance of an optimum quality of life for afflicted individuals and their families. A first step in that direction must be the realization that, despite his or her failing abilities, the person with AD retains some very important skills and, above all, retains those basic psychosocial needs that are common to us all: the needs to be productive, to identify oneself as a valuable individual, and to maintain contact with one's environment and with other people. This is the basis on which the Alzheimer "Day Away" and Home Assistance programs were founded.

It cannot be denied that AD is, thus far, an incurable and ultimately fatal disease. However, the hopeless image of the withdrawn, solitary individual which is so frequently projected of its victims is misleading. Most persons with AD are just as eager to socialize and interact with their environment as is anyone else. They simply lack the skills to do so

independently and spontaneously, and their negative or asocial behavior is usually a consequence of unrealistic expectations and inadequate support systems.

An analogy can be drawn here: It would be foolish to
insist that a one-armed man eat chicken in the conventional
manner, using fork and knife. Equally foolish would be
drawing the conclusion that he is totally incapable of eating
chicken. Imagine his reaction if either of these situations
was presented to him! The humane approach would be to let
him use his fingers or give him an adapted utensil that can
be used with one hand—either way, accommodating his deficits while letting him make full use of his remaining ability.
So, too, persons with Alzheimer's disease cannot be forced
into using resources that they do not have, but they can be
directed toward using fully those resources that they do
retain.

The health care community must counter the fatalistic
attitude that all too often accompanies a diagnosis of AD. It
must continue to develop supportive and therapeutic techniques in the management of AD, draw together resource
networks and facilities to meet the needs of victims, and
take positive action to make these resources available. Persons affected by AD should have access to the type of support systems now afforded to those living with muscular
dystrophy, multiple sclerosis, and other, as yet incurable dis-
eases.

Because AD usually does not produce any overt physical
disability, the extent of the person's handicap and the
resulting stress to his or her family and caregivers may not
always be fully appreciated. Family support, in terms of
counseling, advocacy, and education, is a vital role that the
"Day Away" and Home Assistance programs and the
Alzheimer Society share. It is well known that efforts to
maintain family integrity, ensure the caregiver's physical
and emotional health, and provide the caregiver with effective management techniques have a positive effect on the
client's quality of life. This is another area in which the
health care community must continue to take an active role.

A much-voiced fear among those contemplating a career in working with demented persons and their families is that of "burning out," of being unable to deal with the emotional stress and the depletion of their own personal resources. This fear stems largely from the fatalistic attitude mentioned earlier: the notion that, short of a cure, there are few truly positive contributions to be made. Nothing could be farther from the truth. Programs like "Day Away" and Home Assistance are making use of accumulated clinical knowledge, demonstrating the effectiveness of established techniques, and developing new approaches aimed at maintaining the person with a dementing condition in his or her community for as long and as comfortably as possible.

This work does not end with institutionalization of the client. The concern for maintaining quality of life and satisfying the client's psychosocial needs must continue into the supervised setting.

These are the beginnings in an area where many more positive contributions remain to be made. There are contributions to be made by every level within the community: family practitioners, medical specialists, community and social agency workers, volunteers, workers in supervised housing and institutions, friends, and neighbors all have a role in the process. Their tools may be very sophisticated or very simple. *Doing Things* demonstrates that, used knowledgeably, the very simple activities of daily living can be used as valuable therapeutic tools.

It is hoped that this manual will be used in a dynamic way. The concepts outlined in the preceding pages are just a starting point. As these concepts are shared with colleagues and with clients' families, and as workers incorporate their own experiences and knowledge, ideas will change and grow. After all, doing things is a dynamic process!

Appendix A

In-service for "Day Away" Volunteers

The following in-service seminar was presented to "Day Away" volunteers as part of their training program. It is included here as a model for those planning training sessions within their own facilities.

Objectives

1. Review the intrinsic aims within specific program activities:
   Orientation
   Crafts
   Meal preparation
   Coffee klatch
   Lunch
   Exercise period
2. Review common cognitive problems experienced by many of the clients:
   Initiation
   Sequencing
   Body awareness
   Motor planning
   Judgment

3. Identify techniques that may help clients cope with these impediments.
4. Practice specific skills in guiding clients through to successful completion of the activity:
Verbal guidance
Physical guidance

Objectives as They Relate to Specific Program Activities

Orientation

Confirm time, place, and person
Reestablish membership in the group
Encourage individuals to contribute to the group at a level with which they are comfortable
Explore various themes that are of interest to the group
Prepare for the day's events

Crafts and Other Activities Such as Meal Preparation

Build self-esteem and sense of identity by productive and meaningful activity
Maximize a sense of independence and competence
Provide meaningful sensory stimulation
Explore interests and competencies
Provide a link to past activities wherever this is appropriate
Experience the pleasure of doing

Coffee Klatch and Lunch

Encourage nutrition and fluid intake
Allow comfortable and self-directed social interaction
Practice retained social competencies

Exercise Period

Maintain muscle strength and range of motion
Maintain body awareness through sensation of movement

Provide gentle cardiopulmonary workout
Experience a sense of pleasure and competence in being
    able to follow exercise program and move freely
Encourage group interaction during dance session

Common Cognitive Dysfunctions

Initiation

Clients may have difficulty "getting started," may seem negative or indecisive, may be nervous about not knowing exactly what is expected or where to start. This is common, and they may need specific instructions and concrete clues to help them get started.

Sequencing

Putting actions, events, or objects in a logical order is difficult for many clients. We therefore break the task down into its constituent parts and present one step at a time. This eliminates for clients the need to worry about what comes next and permits them to concentrate fully on the step at hand.

Body Awareness

In order to move smoothly and purposefully, we must have a fairly clear image of how our body is put together, how the various parts are oriented to one another, and how the parts relate to other objects in the environment. When body image becomes diffuse and disorganized, it becomes difficult for the client to call upon specific muscle groups to execute a particular movement accurately.

Motor Planning

This refers to the ability to translate a concept into a movement. It requires the ability to initiate, sequence, and conceptualize one's body position and orientation.

Judgment

Some clients are unable to make accurate judgments about the appropriateness of certain actions or to predict accurately the consequences of certain actions.

Providing Meaningful Guidance and Direction

General Guidelines

- Provide only as much guidance as is necessary for successful completion of the activity within the context of the aims of the activity.
- Keep instructions simple, precise, and consistent with other concrete clues.
- Fade out guidance as soon as the client is on the right track.
- Give reassurance as often as needed, but avoid distracting the client.

Verbal Instructions

- Keep phrases short, with a minimum of extraneous explanation and substantives.
- Give only one step instructions.
- Support verbal instructions with visual clues if possible.
- It often helps to say the client's name to get his/her attention before making a statement.

"Hands-on" Direction

- If you are out of sight of the client, say his/her name and warn him/her that you are going to guide him/her.
- Let your hand rest on the client for a second before you start directing a movement, so he/she can better identify the part to be moved.
- Never persist in moving a totally passive or resistant limb.
- Provide as little manual guidance as is necessary to encourage active movement on the part of the client.

Appendix B

*Occupational Therapy Teaching Sheets
for Caregivers and Sitters*

Appendix B consists of a package that was designed to be used by homemakers and sitters who were working with clients in their homes on days when the clients did not attend "Day Away." It also proved to be an effective means of making the benefits of the program available to clients who for some reason were unable to attend "Day Away."

This package was never intended to be used by the homemaker or sitter in isolation, since it requires the assessment and program planning skills of a trained professional familiar with the needs of AD victims in order to be used effectively.

Alzheimer's disease (AD) is a progressive illness that affects the brain. The most common and obvious symptom is memory loss. However, a person with this disease may also experience difficulties understanding what is said to him/her; expressing himself or herself accurately; planning, organizing, and concentrating on even simple tasks, such as dressing or bathing; finding his/her way around; keeping track of his/her belongings; and recognizing things or people that he/she sees. Since each person is an individual and is affected by the disease differently, securing a therapist's explanation of your client's particular difficulties may be helpful.

The overall effect of the disease is that the person loses the ability to do many of the things that formerly were a normal part of his/her life. This can make a person feel useless and depressed or become frustrated and angry. Since we do not yet know of any cure for AD or any established rehabilitative techniques, our aim is to help the person cope with his/her disability as well as possible. Your regular involvement with that person can be very important in helping him/her stay as active as possible, keep a feeling of self-worth, and stay in touch with the world around him/her.

It is important to keep in mind that even though the person with AD may look quite healthy, he/she is disabled and is dependent on you for accurate, meaningful guidance in order to be able to do things.

General Guidelines

The following are useful principles to remember in interacting with a person who has Alzheimer's disease.

1. Being productive and experiencing a sense of achievement is important to everyone. The person with AD has this need, too. The most common activities of daily living, such as personal hygiene, grooming, food preparation, housekeeping, and simple, familiar pastimes, can be very gratifying accomplishments.

2. The person with AD often has difficulty learning new things, so do not try to teach new skills. Rather, stick to old, familiar activities and ways of doing them. You may be surprised by the things that he/she can do once you get him/her started: for example, cutting pastry dough, paring vegetables, playing the piano, or washing dishes.

3. The person may have difficulty grasping an idea and following through with instructions unless he/she can actually see what you are talking about. For example, "Take out the garbage" may have no meaning to the client if you are sitting with him/her in the living room. If, however, you go

into the kitchen with him/her, show him/her the garbage, and then say, "Let's take it out," he/she will likely be able to do it.

4. Because the person may have difficulty conceptualizing a task and may not be quite sure of what is expected of him/her, he/she may often say "No" when asked if he/she would like to do something. To overcome this, avoid options. Instead of asking the person if he/she wants a sandwich or if he/she wants to go to the washroom, show him/her and tell him/her: "Here is your sandwich"; "You had better go to the washroom before we go out. Come with me."

5. He/she may have difficulty organizing things, solving problems, and anticipating problems. So get things organized. Have all the things you need, and only the things you need, ready before getting him/her involved in an activity. Be prepared to step in and correct a mistake, but do not make an issue of it.

6. You may find that the person needs detailed, step-by-step instructions before he/she can do a task successfully. For example, "Fill the creamer" involves many steps and may need to be broken down into: "Pick up the milk jug"; "Pour it in here" (point to the creamer); "That's enough"; "Put it down."

7. In all your instructions, keep the sentences short and explicit and avoid complicated phrases. Use the same words each time, so that the person gets used to the instructions.

8. Keep your voice calm and at a fairly low pitch. Shouting does not help a person understand and may even make him/her anxious.

9. Support what you are saying with the appropriate body language. Point to things you are talking about. Keep your facial expression consistent with what you are saying. Use touching, such as handshakes, hugs, pats, etc., whenever it is appropriate. Touching the person while you are talking to him/her often helps keep his/her attention.

10. Always talk to the person face to face.

11. It helps to say the person's name at the beginning of a statement to get and keep his/her attention.

12. In your efforts to communicate clearly, though, be careful not to "talk down" to the person or fall into the trap of treating him/her like a child. He/she is, after all, an adult, and is entitled to be treated as such.

13. Make an effort to find out which things the person can do independently and give him/her the opportunity to do these things whenever possible.

14. Memory loss is a big problem to the person with AD, so avoid asking for facts, especially about things that happened recently. Rather, inform him/her about things that have happened. For example, if you go shopping together, review the things you've bought instead of expecting him/her to recall. Be prepared to repeat information frequently, and do it as calmly as if it were the first time you were saying it.

15. Memory of things in the distant past, however, may be quite good and a comfort to the person with AD. Remote memory is often aided with prompts such as photograph albums, keepsakes, or books. Time spent recalling past experiences and accomplishments with the help of such aids can be very fulfilling.

16. Establish a regular routine to your visiting time so that the client need not worry about what is going to happen next and can concentrate on what you are doing now. It will take a while, but if you stick to the routine, it will eventually sink in.

17. Do not be afraid that the routine or repetition of activities will bore the client. Often, the routine provides security, and the repetition of a successful activity gives the client a sense of competence.

Activities

The activities we have found to be most successful with clients who have Alzheimer's disease have been those that are familiar to the client, those that have only one or two steps that can be repeated over and over again, and those that have an obvious purpose and outcome. Many complex activities, such as preparing a meal or doing a load of laundry, include components in which the client can participate. The following are examples of various activities that may be helpful in planning the routine of your visit. They may not all be appropriate for the client with whom you are involved. If you have any doubts, please consult the occupational therapist. Nor is this list all inclusive. You may be able to add ideas stemming from your own knowledge of the client.

Household chores provide familiar tasks that promote a sense of achievement and keep a person in touch with his/her immediate surroundings.

Dusting, sweeping, mopping, polishing furniture
Laundry: sorting, hanging, folding
Washing or drying dishes
Watering or transplanting plants
Raking leaves
Sorting out drawers and closets

Self-care activities build self-esteem, a positive self-image, and sense of independence.

Dressing
Grooming: combing hair, caring for skin, getting a
    manicure, applying make-up, going to the beauty parlor
    (The client may not be able to perform these tasks
    independently, but he/she can still be involved by
    looking in the mirror, watching the manicure, choosing
    colors and styles, etc.)
Eating meals and snacks

Meal preparation involves familiar activities that have a positive outcome that is appreciable by others as well as by self. Sensory experiences of smell and taste can be encouraged.

Chopping, cleaning, paring, peeling fruit and vegetables for
    casseroles, sauces, sandwiches, salads, side dishes, etc.
Cutting pastry or cookies
Stirring, kneading, mixing

Grating cheese or vegetables, etc.
Setting the table

Outings promote physical activity, help the client keep in touch with the community, and offer stimulation outside the home. It is best to avoid crowded, overstimulating places.

Walks to buy regular items such as newspaper or milk
(Buying a little something that is special, such as a plant or a tube of lipstick, also lifts spirits.)
Walks to the park to watch children in playground, etc.
(Point out flowers, trees, and other sights. Comment on changes in the neighborhood.)
Window shopping (In winter, covered malls are good. Pet stores, car showrooms, florists, plant nurseries, and markets, all are fun.)
"Freebies" (Some jewelers, for example, offer free cleaning of rings. Clients enjoy doing this from time to time.)
Bus rides
Coffee at a coffee shop
Museums, art galleries, exhibits when available

Crafts tap old skills and provide comfort and a sense of achievement.

Clients who used to knit, crochet, or embroider may still be able to do simple stitching to edge napkins, knit or crochet granny squares or scarves, or knit the tube part of socks. It is rarely effective to introduce a new craft with which the client was not familiar in the past, unless it is very simple. Another concern is that if the client is left unattended with the craft activity between your visits, he/she may try to continue independently and may inadvertently spoil the project. This would be very disappointing. If you do start a project, it may be best to put it away between visits and reserve it for the times you spend with the client.

Quiet activities and reminiscence permit the client to recall important events and interests from the past.

Listening to favorite music

Looking through books, magazines, picture albums,
cookbooks (Since many clients find it difficult to
understand printed material, it is best to use books with
many pictures.)

Sorting through keepsakes

Program Plan

The following areas are filled out by the therapist in con-
junction with the homemaker. Where appropriate, the client
is included in the discussion.

Sample Objectives

1. Improve self-esteem
2. Maintain adequate nutrition
3. Maintain contact with the community
4. Maintain involvement in household activities

Sample Methods

Related to objective number 1: Select one activity daily that
relates to grooming.

Related to objective number 2: With client, prepare a
nutritious dinner that he/she can eat later.

Related to objective number 3: Include a walk outdoors each
day; buy a newspaper and read selected items with client
each visit.

Related to objective number 4: Involve the client in one
specific household task each day.

Daily Plan

The daily plan sheet can be very helpful for the homemaker.
In designing a daily plan, the homemaker should keep in
mind that the sequence, not precise timing, is important.

The following partial sheet has been filled in as an
example.

Time	Type of Activity	Options
10:00	Activity 1 introduction and plan for the day	make tea and chat about things to do
10:30	Activity 2 housekeeping	clean refrigerator dust furniture vacuum sort clothes (choose one)
11:00	Activity 3 prepare lunch	soup sandwiches desert
11:45	Activity 4 eat lunch	
12:15	Activity 5 clear dishes	clear table wash dishes dry dishes put dishes away (assign 2 jobs to client)
12:30	Activity 6	

Communication Sheet

Through this written record, the supervising therapist can keep in touch with the activities of the homemaker and the client. It also serves as a record for the homemaker of activities that have been successful and those that have not. It will be the basis upon which the therapist and the homemaker develop additional program ideas.

Date	Activities	Outcome	Signature

Appendix C

Evaluation Protocol

NAME: _MRS. JANE DOE_

INITIAL OBSERVATIONS
APPARENT AGE: _AS STATED_   APPARENT HEALTH _GOOD_

GROOMING: _GOOD_   DRESS: _GOOD_   POSTURE: _O.K._   GAIT: _SLOW_

MOVEMENTS: _SLOW_   ACTIVITY LEVEL: _REDUCED_   AFFECT: _APPROPRIATE_

BEHAVIOR
TOWARD INTERVIEWER: _HESITANT BUT COURTEOUS_

TOWARD CAREGIVER: _DEPENDENT - LOOKED TO HER OFTEN FOR HELP_

LIVING CONDITIONS
TYPE OF DWELLING: _2-STORY SINGLE FAMILY_   No. OCCUPANTS _6_

RELATIONSHIP TO CLIENT: _DAUGHTER, SON-IN-LAW, 2 GRANDSONS_

CONDITION OF DWELLING: _EXCELLENT_

LENGTH OF OCCUPANCY: _FAMILY - 5 YEARS, CLIENT - 6 WEEKS_

REGULAR CONTACTS: _OUTSIDE IMMEDIATE FAMILY - 2 SISTERS CALL_

ACCESSIBLE FACILITIES IN THE COMMUNITY: _SHOPPING AREA_

CLIENT'S METHOD OF ACCESSING COMMUNITY FACILITIES: _DAUGHTER_

  OBSTACLES TO ACCESS: _CLIENT'S FEAR OF GETTING LOST_

CLIENT'S FAMILIARITY WITH DWELLING: _CANNOT FIND THINGS_

CLIENT'S FAMILIARITY WITH COMMUNITY: _POOR_

EVIDENT HAZARDS IN THE HOME: _NONE - AS CLIENT TAKES FEW INITIATIVES_

EVIDENT HAZARDS IN THE COMMUNITY: _CLIENT DOES NOT VENTURE_

POTENTIAL HAZARDS: _CLIENT IS ALONE IN HOUSE 2-3 HOURS DAILY_

DO UNFAMILIAR PERSONS COME TO THE HOME REGULARLY? _PAPER CARRIER_

CLIENT'S AWARENESS OF HAZARDS: _VERBALIZES AWARENESS_

SOCIAL HISTORY

ETHNIC ORIGIN: _FRENCH CANADIAN_ RELIGIOUS AFFILIATION: _K/C_

MOTHER TONGUE: _FRENCH_ LANGUAGE NOW SPOKEN: _FRENCH_

PLACE OF BIRTH: _QUEBEC CITY_ FATHER'S OCCUPATION: _TRADESMAN_

No. SIBLINGS: _3 SISTERS_ LOCATIONS: _1 DECEASED ; 2 IN AYLMER_

EDUCATION: _GRADE 8_

OCCUPATIONS: _KEYPUNCH OPERATOR_

MARITAL STATUS: _WIDOWED_ No. CHILDREN: _1 DAUGHTER_

LOCATION OF CHILDREN: _CLIENT LIVES WITH ONLY DAUGHTER_

HOBBIES, CLUBS AND INTERESTS, PAST: _SEWING, KNITTING, DANCING_

PRESENT: _T.V._

FINANCES: Pension? _YES_ Medicare? _NO_ Blue Cross/Blue Shield? _NO_

LEGAL: POWER OF ATTORNEY? _NO - HAS JOINT ACCOUNT WITH DAUGHTER_

INFORMATION ON FAMILY SUPPORT GIVEN? _YES_ INTEREST SHOWN? _YES_

HEALTH HISTORY

GENERAL HEALTH OF CLIENT: _GOOD - HAS DIFFICULTY SWALLOWING_
INVESTIGATED BY DOCTOR - RESULTS NEGATIVE

GENERAL HEALTH OF CAREGIVER: _GOOD - EMOTIONALLY STRESSED BY NEW_
BURDEN, NEED TO LEAVE JOB, AND MARITAL STRESS RE MOTHER

SPECIALISTS INVOLVED: _DR. SMITH - NEUROLOGIST_ PHONE: _569-3950_
DR. JONES - PSYCHOLOGIST PHONE: _631-7950_

MEDICATIONS: _ANTIACID P.R.N._ DIET: _NORMAL - AVOIDS_
HALIDOL P.R.N. _DRY FOODS_

ALLERGIES: _NONE_

COMPLIANCE WITH HEALTH RESTRICTIONS: _REFUSES ALL PILLS_

VISION: _GOOD_ GLASSES: _READING_ HEARING: _AIDED_ HEARING AID: R _✓_ L __

MOBILITY AIDS USED: _NONE_

DIAGNOSTIC PROCEDURE FOR AD USED: _CAT SCAN EEG NEUROPSYCH_

WHEN AND HOW DID FAMILY FIRST NOTICE THE PROBLEM? _3 YEARS GRADUAL_
DECLINE IN ABILITY TO CARE FOR SELF, LANGUAGE PROBLEMS NOTICED 1 YEAR AGO

ACTIVITIES OF DAILY LIVING

TASK	INDEPEND-ENT	WITH ERRORS	WITH SU-PERVISION	WITH HELP	DEPEND-ENT
TOILETING	YES			ONLY WITH TIGHT CLOTHES	
GROOMING				COULD DO	BUT DAUGHTER DOES ALL
DRESSING		SEQUENCING & MATCHING COLOURS			
UNDRESSING	YES				
BATHING			TO WASH PROPERLY	IN AND OUT OF TUB	
FEEDING	YES	USES WRONG UTENSIL			
MOBILITY IN THE HOME	GOOD				
WALKING	GOOD				
USE OF PUBLIC TRANSPORTATION					NEVER DOES
FOOD PREPARATION				COULD HELP	NEVER DOES
HOUSEKEEPING				LIGHT CHORES	
MONEY MANAGEMENT					NEVER DOES
TAKING MEDICATIONS					REFUSES
TELEPHONE ANSWERING		BECOMES ANXIOUS			
TELEPHONE CALLING					NEVER DOES
RECREATION					

NUTRITION:
SAMPLE MENU: *BALANCED DIET PROVIDED BY DAUGHTER*

TIME USE:
SAMPLE ROUTINE: *INSISTS ON ROUTINE*

TASK ORIENTATION:
(ask client to make a cup of tea): *BECAME VERY ANXIOUS - BUT DID WITH STEP-BY-STEP INSTRUCTIONS*

NAME: *JANE DOE*

EXPRESSIVE LANGUAGE

GENERAL QUALITY OF CONVERSATION (superficial, disjointed, etc.)

GENERALLY CONCRETE, SUPERFICIAL, AND REPETITIVE

INITIATES: *SELDOM* ___ RESPONDS ONLY: *USUALLY*

FAILS TO EXPRESS COMPLETE THOUGHT: *YES* ___ LOSES TOPIC: *YES*

USES SINGLE WORDS: *NO* ___ USES COMPLETE SENTENCES: *LONG*

CIRCUMLOCUTION: *YES* PARAPHASIAS: *YES* INTRUSION: *NO* ECHOLALIA: *NO*

(ask client to name) PENCIL: *PENCIL* WATCH: *TIME* CHAIR: *CHAIR*

(ask client to name parts) LEAD: *WRITE* HAND: *NO* ___ LEG: *NO*

RECEPTIVE LANGUAGE

(ask client to) "CLOSE YOUR EYES AND TOUCH YOUR LEFT EAR": *O.K*

(ask client to read and follow commands)

"OPEN YOUR MOUTH": *READ ALOUD BUT COULD NOT PERFORM ACTION*

"CLOSE YOUR EYES AND TOUCH YOUR LEFT EAR": *READ BUT DID NOT DO*

PERCEPTUAL-MOTOR FUNCTION

GROSS MOTOR COORDINATION: *O.K.* ___ RHYTHM: *IMPAIRED*

BALANCE: WALKING: *O.K.* ___ STANDING: *O.K* ___ SITTING: *O.K*

NAVIGATION: DOES THE CLIENT BUMP INTO OBSTACLES? *NO*

FINE MOTOR COORDINATION (stand pencil on end): *TRIED*

EYE-HAND COORDINATION (trace ◇): *HAD DIFFICULTY WITH CORNERS*

PROPRIOCEPTION (touch nose with eyes closed): *MISSED BY ONE INCH*

BIMANUAL COORDINATION (place cap on pen): *GOOD*

(screw nut onto bolt): *COULD NOT TURN NUT*

ADDITIONAL OBSERVATIONS

CLIENT HAS MUCH DIFFICULTY WITH MOTOR PLANNING. SHE BECOMES FRUSTRATED AND GIVES UP. SHE IS VERY RELUCTANT TO TRY UNFAMILIAR TASKS.

COGNITIVE ABILITIES

JUDGMENT AND INSIGHT

CLIENT'S PERCEPTION OF HIS OWN CAPABILITIES AND LIMITATIONS: *ADMITS TO POOR MEMORY. CLAIMS SHE CAN DO NOTHING*

EVIDENT LIMITATIONS DENIED BY CLIENT: *N/A*

NAME: _JANE DOE_

(ask client)

"WHAT WOULD YOU DO IF THERE WERE A FIRE IN THE HOUSE?"
GET OUT

"IF YOU WERE LOST IN THE STREET?" _ASK SOME ONE_

"IF A STRANGER CAME TO THE DOOR?" _DON'T OPEN DOOR_

(ask client to explain a proverb, e.g.)

"A ROLLING STONE GATHERS NO MOSS" _NO IDEA_

(ask the client to identify)

WHAT IS SIMILAR ABOUT A PIG AND A CAT? _PIG IS PIG_

PANTS AND A DRESS? _ONE FOR MEN; ONE WOMEN_

A BANANA AND AN ORANGE? _ONE IS YELLOW; OTHER, ORANGE_

ORIENTATION

(does client know) THE DATE? _NO_ THE DAY? _NO_ THE MONTH? _NO_

THE YEAR? _NO_ SEASON? _NO_ TIME OF DAY? _YES_ PLACE? _YES_ CITY? _NO_

MEMORY

LONG TERM (ask client)

NAMES OF HIS/HER CHILDREN _LIVES WITH ONLY DAUGHTER_

PLACE OF OWN BIRTH _NO_

FATHER'S OCCUPATION _NO_

NO. OF GRANDCHILDREN _LIVES WITH ONLY TWO_

REGISTRATION (Show client 5 familiar objects. Which ones can he/she recall immediately after they are removed?)

1. _SPOON_ 2. _—_ 4. _—_ 5. _—_

LEARNING (number of trials to recall 3 of the above): _2 AFTER 3 TRIALS_

RECENT MEMORY (number of objects recalled after 5 minutes): _0_

(omit the following if doing H.D.S.)

PRAXIS (ask client to imitate hand postures)

SINGLE RING: _YES_ DOUBLE RING: _NO_ REVERSE HANDS: _NO_

(ask client to demonstrate use of)

IMAGINARY COMB: _NO_ IMAGINARY HAMMER: _NO_ IMAGINARY CANDLE: _NO_

CONCENTRATION

(ask client to)   COUNT 10-1: _YES_

COUNT 63-50: _NO_

RECITE DAYS OF THE WEEK BACKWARD: _NO_

124

CALCULATION

$2 + 1 =$ _3_ $4 - 2 =$ _2_ $12 + 4 =$ _?_ $53 + 17 =$ _?_

VISUAL ATTENTION

FIND ONE ITEM IN COMPLEX PICTURE: _DISCUSSED WHOLE PICTURE_

CONSTRUCTION

COPY TOOTHPICK SQUARE: _NO- BECAME VERY FRUSTRATED_

BODY IMAGE

KNOWS: BODY PARTS ON SELF: _YES_

BODY PARTS ON INTERVIEWER: _YES_

LEFT & RIGHT ON SELF: _YES_

LEFT & RIGHT ON INTERVIEWER: _NO_

WRITING

SIGNATURE (do on back of sheet & comment here): _1ST NAME ONLY_

SENTENCE (do on back of sheet & comment here): _SEVERAL LETTERS ONLY_

ADDITIONAL COMMENTS

CLIENT WAS NEVER CERTAIN IF SHE HAD GIVEN THE CORRECT RESPONSE AND OFTEN ASKED HER DAUGHTER FOR HELP

SUMMARY

OVERALL DEGREE OF IMPAIRMENT: _MODERATE TO SEVERE_

CLIENT'S MAJOR STRENGTHS: _BASIC HABITUAL SKILLS, SOCIAL SKILLS_

CLIENT'S MAJOR DEFICITS: _MEMORY, MOTOR PLANNING, LANGUAGE_

MAJOR COMPENSATORY MECHANISMS AND SUPPORTS USED BY

CLIENT: _SOCIAL ABILITY AND DEPENDENCE ON DAUGHTER_

CAREGIVER: _DESIRE TO DO BEST FOR MOTHER - FOSTERS DEPENDENCE_

MAJOR PROBLEMS IDENTIFIED BY FAMILY: _LACK OF PRIVACY_

FAMILY'S FEELINGS ABOUT PLACEMENT: _WISH TO DELAY AS LONG AS POSSIBLE_

FAMILY'S EXPECTATIONS OF "DAY AWAY": _RESPITE, SOCIAL STIMULATION_

OF HOME ASSISTANCE: _SAW NO NEED_

CLIENT'S FEELINGS ABOUT "DAY AWAY": _APPREHENSIVE, WILLING TO TRY_

ABOUT HOME ASSISTANCE: _NOT DISCUSSED_

IMPRESSIONS: *THIS LADY HAD BEEN LIVING ON HER OWN WHILE VERY HANDICAPPED AND THEREFORE MUST HAVE BEEN VERY STRESSED. SHE IS REACTING TO HER NEW SITUATION BY BECOMING TOTALLY DEPENDENT. PSYCHOMOTOR RETARDATION MAY ALSO SUGGEST PRESENCE OF DEPRESSION.*

PLANS AND RECOMMENDATIONS:

- *ENROLL IN FRENCH "DAY AWAY" GROUP AS SOON AS POSSIBLE.*
- *IDENTIFY SPECIFIC TASKS AND RECREATIONAL ACTIVITIES WHICH MRS. DOE CAN DO AND ENJOY AND TYPE OF ASSISTANCE SHE NEEDS TO SUCCEED.*
- *DEMONSTRATE THESE TO FAMILY AND SUPPORT THEM IN FOLLOWING THROUGH WITH APPROPRIATE ONES AT HOME.*
- *ENCOURAGE FAMILY TO ATTEND FAMILY SUPPORT GROUPS.*
- *REFER TO PSYCHIATRIST FOR EVALUATION RE POSSIBLE DEPRESSION.*

SIGNATURE: *Mary Jones*

DATE: *MARCH 15, 1986*

Activity Program Plan for Jane Doe

Strengths

Ability to perform basic habitual skills
Good social skills
Ability to follow simple step-by-step instructions
Good mobility
Good primary motor skills

Weaknesses

Language problems hinder communication with unfamiliar
    people
Poor motor planning ability
Poor recent memory
Disorientation in relation to time and place causes anxiety
Lack of confidence in existing skills, and reluctance to try

Needs

Socialization
Self-esteem from successful experience

Methods

Include Jane actively in social activities.

Minimize pressure on Jane to express herself verbally, and provide appropriate cues and supports when she has difficulty.

Include Jane in gross motor activities, especially dancing, which is an old skill.

Include Jane in group projects as an observer at first to give her an opportunity to practice her social strengths and gain confidence before trying the activity.

Use one-step repetitive activities (e.g., painting Podgy, chopping, sanding).

Encourage useful household tasks (e.g., dusting furniture, folding towels, and dishwashing) and through journal encourage follow-through at home.

Encourage grooming, especially manicure, hair, and make-up, to improve self-image.

Give step-by-step instruction in more complex tasks.

Encourage active participation in orientation discussion of date and place. Reinforce this often throughout the day.

Address Jane from the right side (hearing aid).

Notes

Introduction

1. Nancy L. Mace and Peter V. Rabins, *A Survey of Day Care for the Demented Adult in the United States* (Washington, D.C.: National Council on Aging, 1984).
2. Frances Hadley and Anne Opzoomer, " 'Day Away,' a Community Based Program for the Alzheimer Victim" (Paper presented at the Eleventh Annual Meeting of the Ontario Psychogeriatric Association, Toronto, Ontario, 1984).
3. Kenneth E. Mobily and Thea M. Horft, "The Family's Dilemma: Alzheimer's Disease," *Activities, Adaptations, and Aging* 6, no. 4 (1985): 63–71.

Chapter 1

1. Joseph T. Coyle, "On Senility, Alzheimer's Disease, and the Cholinergic Link," *Executive Health* 29 (March 1983): 6.
2. Robert J. Joynt and Ira Shoulson, "Dementia," in *Clinical Neuropsychology,* ed. Kenneth H. Heilman and Edward Valenstein, 2d ed. (New York: Oxford University Press, 1985).
3. Ibid.
4. Guy Proulx, "Brain and Behavior" (Lecture delivered at "Day Away" in-service, September 1985).
5. Ibid.
6. Ibid.

7. V. A. Krag, "Senescent Forgetfulness: Benign and Malignant," *Canadian Medical Association Journal* 86, no. 6 (1962): 257–61.

8. Proulx, "Brain and Behavior."

9. Ibid.

10. Joynt and Shoulson, "Dementia."

11. Joseph G. Chusio and Joseph J. McDonald, *Correlative Neuroanatomy and Functional Neurology,* 12th ed. (Los Altos, Calif.: Lange Medical Publications 1964).

12. Joynt and Shoulson, "Dementia."

13. Chusio and McDonald, *Correlative Neuroanatomy.*

14. Kenneth M. Heilman and Leslie J. Ganzalez Roth, "Apraxia," in *Clinical Neuropsychology,* ed. Heilman and Valenstein.

15. Joynt and Shoulson, "Dementia."

Chapter 2

1. W. B. Dalziel, personal communication, March 1986.

2. Ibid.

3. G. McKhann, D. Drachman, M. Folstein et al., "Clinical Diagnosis of Alzheimer's Disease: Report of the NINCDS-ADRDA Work Group under the Auspices of the Department of Health and Human Services Task Force on Alzheimer's Disease," *Neurology* 34 (1984): 939–44.

4. Kerry Hamsher, "Mental Status Examination in Alzheimer's Disease: The Neuropsychologist's Role," *Postgraduate Medicine* 73, no. 4 (1983): 225–28.

5. McKhann, Drachman, Folstein et al., "Clinical Diagnosis of Alzheimer's Disease."

6. Albert A. Fisk, "Management of Alzheimer's Disease," *Postgraduate Medicine* 73, no. 4 (1983): 237–41.

7. Mary Ninos and Rennie Makohon, "Functional Assessment of the Patient," *Geriatric Nursing* 6, no. 3 (1985): 139–42.

8. M. G. Cole, D. P. Dastoor, and D. Koszych, "The Hierarchic Dementia Scale," *Journal of Clinical Experimental Gerontology* 5, no. 3 (1983): 219–34.

9. J. Zarit and S. Zarit, "Measuring Burden and Support in Families with Alzheimer's Disease Elders" (Paper delivered at the Thirty-fifth Annual Meeting of the Gerontological Society of America, 1982).

Chapter 3

1. Jacqueline S. Edelson and Walter Lyons, *Institutional Care of the Mentally Impaired Elderly* (New York: Van Nostrand Reinhold, 1985).
2. J. R. Phillips, "Music in the Nursing of Elderly Persons in Nursing Homes," *Journal of Gerontologic Nursing* 6, no. 1 (1980): 37–39.
3. Enid J. Portnoy, "Reminiscence Is a Valuable Communication Tool for the Elderly," *Geriatric Care* 17, no. 6 (1985).

Chapter 4

1. Abraham Maslow, *Motivation and Personality,* 2d ed. (New York: Harper and Row, 1970).

Glossary

Affect The outward manifestation of a person's feelings, usually referring to facial expression and posture.

Aggression A forceful, attacking action; may be physical or verbal and may be directed at people or at objects.

Agnosia The inability, in the absence of any direct impairment of the sensory organs, to recognize familiar stimuli experienced by means of the senses. This inability may be related to any of the senses: sight, hearing, touch, smell, and taste. Visual, auditory, and tactile agnosias, however, are most common.

Alexia A disturbance in the ability to read. Primary ALEXIA is related to visual AGNOSIA, whereas secondary ALEXIA is due to deficits in language. Many victims of AD can read aloud fluently but have no comprehension of the material they are reading.

Anomia The inability to recall the correct word or phrase to express an intended thought or to identify a familiar object accurately.

Aphasia A deficit or loss of the ability to express oneself by means of speech or the written word in the absence of any muscular or intellectual impairment.

Apraxia The inability to carry out skilled and purposeful movements in the absence of any physical impairment or paralysis.

Body Image The knowledge of how one's body looks, how it is organized, and how the various parts of it relate to one another. Accurate body image is essential for comfortable movement through space; for dressing, bathing, and grooming; and for most other activities of daily life.

Catastrophic Reaction An excessively anxious, fearful, or despairing reaction to frustration resulting from an individual's inability to perform a task or understand a situation.

Circumlocution "Talking around the issue," a characteristic of speech common to persons suffering from ANOMIA. In their effort to express a thought or identify an object, they describe it by its use, location, or other characteristics.

Cognitive Functions The intellectual processes by which one becomes aware of, perceives, expresses, and understands ideas. These functions involve all aspects of perception, memory, reasoning, and language.

Computerized Axial Tomography (CAT) Scan A type of X-ray investigation that provides a series of detailed sectional images of structures. It is used to identify the presence of tumors, infarcts (dead or damaged brain tissue resulting from strokes), bone displacements, and brain atrophy (shrinking).

Confusion Bewilderment and lack of orderly thought and reactions based on fact. Also the inability to act and choose decisively.

Cortex The outer layer of a body organ. The brain's outer layer is called the cerebral cortex. It is most highly developed in humans and is the seat of higher intellectual functions. It is the part of the brain that is primarily affected by the process of Alzheimer's disease.

Delirium An acute episode of confusion and disorientation.

Delusion A persistent but untrue belief or perception that is held by the person even though it is illogical and not real.

Dementia A progressive and chronic deterioration in cognitive functions resulting from organic brain disorder and usually accompanied by impaired memory and judgment, impulsive behavior, and personality changes. This condition is sometimes confused with *delirium*, which is usually associated with an acute illness or physical disorder, such as malnutrition, dehydration, drug toxicity, or fever, and is usually treatable and reversible. Untreated delirium may lead to chronic dementia.

Disorientation The lack of accurate knowledge concerning time, place, one's identity, and/or the identity of familiar others. The lack of knowledge regarding the purpose of events may also be included in this definition.

Echolalia Automatic and often persistent repetition of words and/or expressions just heard by the individual; acting as an echo.

Electroencephalograph (EEG) A diagnostic tool that measures the quality and quantity of electrical activity in the brain. In Alzheimer's disease, E.E.G. readings may be abnormal.

Hallucinations Sensory perceptions that are not the result of external stimuli. They may affect any of the senses and they are very real to the affected person but to no one else. They are frequently confused with *illusions*.

Illusions Misperceptions that result in a mistaken impression about things. Everyone experiences illusions at one time or another, but they occur with more frequency to people with impaired perceptual abilities.

Inertia The inability to begin a task or initiate a movement in the absence of a concrete stimulus.

Intrusion The persistence of a previous idea or concept to the point where it interferes and "intrudes" on present thoughts or actions. For example: following a discussion about a tree, an individual is asked to name three unassociated objects. The word *tree* may continue to interfere with the individual's ability to respond accurately to the task at hand.

Memory The ability to store, retain, and retrieve information experienced through the senses.

Motor Planning The ability to conceptualize, organize, and carry out a particular series of movements toward a specific end.

Paraphasia The use of an inappropriate word to express a thought or identify an object or person. Although the person's intention is correct, the wrong word comes out.

Perception The ability to interpret accurately and correctly information received through the senses.

Perseveration The persistent repetition of an action associated with the inability to stop unless an outside force intervenes.

Praxis The ability to carry out skilled, organized movements.

Receptive Aphasia The inability, in the absence of sensory or intellectual impairment, to understand spoken or written language.

Sequencing The ability to place things, events, or actions into a logical order so as to arrive at the desired end. Most multistep tasks require accurate sequencing if the outcome is to be successful.

Spatial Orientation The ability to know where one is in space and relative to objects in one's environment. Also the ability to perceive how objects relate to one another, either in front, behind, on, under, to the left, or to the right. It is associated with *directionality,* which is an appreciation of movement toward, away from, to the left, to the right, upward, downward.

Annotated Bibliography

The following materials will be of interest to those involved in programs for demented clients in both institutional and community facilities. The materials are listed here under three headings: Help for the Client, Help for the Family, and Community Programs. Many of the works overlap the boundaries of these categories, but in each case placement was determined by the predominant theme.

Help for the Client

Ackermann, Joan. "Separated, Not Isolated: As Basic as Administrative, Backing, and Commitment." *Journal of Long-Term Care Administration* 13, no. 3 (1985): 91–94.

Describes the institution of a special nursing unit at St. Joseph's Hospital in Yonkers, New York, which addresses the special needs of residents with Alzheimer's disease and related disorders. Specifically describes the environmental and attitudinal accommodations made to maintain the residents' comfort and functional level.

Bartol, Mari Anne. "Nonverbal Communication in Patients with Alzheimer's Disease." *Journal of Gerontological Nursing* 5, no. 4 (1979): 21–31.

Stresses the importance of body language in communicating with mentally impaired clients.

The Burke Rehabilitation Center. *Managing the Person with Intellectual Loss (Dementia or Alzheimer's Disease) at Home.* White Plains, N.Y., 1985.

Provides practical alternatives to the most common problems experienced by caregivers of a demented person living at home. Many of the solutions suggested in this booklet are applicable in the day care setting, as well.

Burnside, Irene Motenson. "Alzheimer's Disease: An Overview." *Journal of Gerontological Nursing* 5, no. 4 (1979): 14–20.

An overview of nursing and medical literature related to Alzheimer's disease and therapeutic considerations. Bibliography is outdated but textual information remains valid.

Cohen, Donna, et al. "Phases of Change in the Patient with Alzheimer's Dementia: A Conceptual Dimension for Defining Health Care Management." *Journal of the American Geriatrics Society* 32, no. 1 (1984): 11–15.

Describes the emotional processes experienced by the patient faced with a progressive dementia and identifies the supports needed at the various stages of the disease.

Coons, Dorothy. "Alive and Well at Wesley Hall." *O.A.H.A. Quarterly,* July 1985.

Describes an in-patient program especially designed for patients with Alzheimer's disease. The environmental accommodations made and the attention given to the patients' needs are applicable to any facility serving this population.

Cox, Kim G. "Milieu Therapy." *Geriatric Nursing* 6, no. 3 (1985): 152–54.

Describes the participation of eight patients in the early to moderately severe stages of Alzheimer's disease in a study using group activities within a therapeutic milieu. The objective was to help patients build a sense of dignity and strengthen existing coping strategies in dealing with their disease.

Edelson, Jacqueline S., and Walter Lyons. *Institutional Care of the Mentally Impaired Elderly.* New York: Van Nostrand Reinhold, 1985.

Sensitively written, this book covers many aspects of the interpersonal care of the mentally impaired resident. Especially recommended.

Fisk, Albert A. "Management of Alzheimer's Disease." *Postgraduate Medicine* 73, no. 4 (1983): 237–41.

Identifies the role of the physician in helping the client and the family cope with diagnosis and the subsequent management problems. Also describes briefly a day program for AD clients.

Geriatric Care. Reno, Nev.: Eymann Publications.

A monthly publication in newsletter format intended "especially for those who care for and about the aging." Available from the publisher at 1490 Huntington Circle, Box 3577, Reno, Nevada 89505. Extremely worthwhile.

Goodwin, Dennis. *The Activity Director's Treasure Chest.* Kissimmee, Fl. The Activity Factory.

Offers effective activity ideas related to clients' needs. Available from the publisher at 1551 Key Court, Kissimmee, Florida 32743.

Haugen, Kristian. "Behavior of Patients with Dementia." *Danish Medical Bulletin* 32, no. 1 (1985): 62–65.

Focuses on the social and psychological factors that influence the behavior of demented patients and identifies therapeutic measures related to orientation, socialization, and environmental design.

Mace, Nancy, and Peter Rabins. *The 36-Hour Day: A Family Guide to Caring for Persons with Alzheimer's Disease, Related Dementing Illnesses, and Memory Loss in Later Life.* Baltimore: Johns Hopkins University Press, 1981.

Provides caregivers practical information and support in all aspects of caring for a person with memory loss.

Ontario Association of Homes for the Aged. *Does It Really Matter If It's Tuesday? A Guide to Caring for the Mentally Impaired Elderly.* Woodbridge, Ontario.

A selection of readings related to care for the mentally impaired elderly. Available from the association at 8 Director Court, Suites 201–202, Woodbridge, Ontario, Canada L4L 3Z5.

Rathbone-McCuan, Eloise, and Joan Hashimi. "Alzheimer's Disease and Isolation." In *Isolated Elders,* 272–305. Rockville, Md.: Aspen Systems, 1982.

Identifies the isolating effects of Alzheimer's disease. Includes case studies and research, along with proposed social systems that could address the needs of clients and their families.

Reisberg, Barry. "Stages of Cognitive Decline." *American Journal of Nursing* 84, no. 2 (1984): 225–28.

A very practical article outlining the various stages of Alzheimer's disease in terms of observable manifestations, impact on the family, and implications for professional care.

Ricci, Marilyn. "All-Out Care for the Alzheimer Patient." *Geriatric Nursing* 4, no. 6 (1983): 369–71.

One nurse's four years of work in a one-on-one program with a lady in the total-care unit has not improved the resident's level of function but has contributed much to her quality of life and has taught a great deal to the staff and family involved. Outlines many one-on-one activities and environmental modifications which proved successful with a severely impaired resident.

Roach, Marion. "Reflection in a Fatal Mirror." *Discover* 6, no. 8 (1985): 76–85.

Describes Barry Reisberg's model of Alzheimer's disease as retrograde development. Gives insight into the behaviors observed in patients. This model is used positively to help prolong maximum function.

Tariot, Pierre, et al. "How Memory Fails: A Theoretical Model." *Geriatric Nursing* 6, no. 3 (1985): 144–47.

Offers a theoretical model for the specific nature of memory loss in Alzheimer's disease and suggests management techniques that enable patients to retain their functional abilities.

Yoe, Mary Ruth. "Dementia." *Johns Hopkins Magazine* 33, no. 6 (1982): 23–30.

Gives insight into the work done by Peter Rabins and Nancy Mace at the Johns Hopkins Medical Center Psychogeriatric Unit. Also describes their approach to clients and their families.

Help for the Family

Eisdorfer, Carl, and Donna Cohen. "Management of the Patient and Family Coping with Dementing Illness." *Journal of Family Practice* 12, no. 5 (1981): 831–37.

Directed mainly to clinicians, this article also identifies important considerations in helping families plan changes in their lifestyle which may facilitate the care of their loved one at home.

Gwyther, Lisa P., and Mary Ann Matteson. "Care for the Caregivers." *Journal of Gerontological Nursing* 9, no. 2 (1983): 93–95.

Outlines the effects on the family of each of the stages of the disease and suggests ways in which support workers can be of help.

La Vargna, Donna. "Group Treatment for Wives of Patients with Alzheimer's Disease." *Social Work and Health Care* 5, no. 2 (1979): 219–21.

Gives a sensitive insight into the feelings of women whose husbands are afflicted by a dementing disease.

Mobily, Kenneth E., and Thea M. Hoeft. "The Family's Dilemma: Alzheimer's Disease." *Activities, Adaptations and Aging* 6, no. 4 (1984): 63–71.

Stresses the importance of leisure, counseling, exercise, and meditation and of maintaining the focus on the things clients can do rather than on the things they cannot do.

Rabins, Peter V. "Management of Dementia in the Family Context." *Psychosomatics* 25, no. 5 (1984).

Identifies problems and loss of skills experienced by the client which are often unknown to the family and which result in interpersonal problems. Discusses the difficulty family members have in coping with conflicting roles and responsibilities.

Safford, Florence. "A Program for Families of the Mentally Impaired Elderly." *Gerontologist* 20, no. 6 (1980): 656–60.

Describes a group program for caregivers. Especially useful in identifying many of the interpersonal problems caregivers experience in interacting with their mentally impaired relative.

Teusink, Paul J. "Helping Families Cope with Alzheimer's Disease." *Hospital and Community Psychiatry* 35, no. 2 (1984): 152–56.

Describes a five-stage reaction process undergone by families facing a progressive, debilitating disease and identifies specific problems faced by these families.

Community Programs

Aronson, Miriam K., et al. "A Community-Based Family/Patient Group Program for Alzheimer's Disease." *Gerontologist* 24, no. 4 (1984): 339–42.

A brief description of a weekly family/patient group established in New York. The bulk of the discussion centers around the family support group and its objectives.

Keyes, Barbara, and Greg Szpak. "Day Care." *Postgraduate Medicine* 73, no. 4 (1983): 245–50.

A brief description of a day program for persons with Alzheimer's disease which was established in Wisconsin. The family support component is described in detail.

Sands, Dan, and Thelma Suzuki. "Adult Day Care for Alzheimer's Patients and Their Families." *Gerontologist* 23, no. 1 (1981): 21–23.

Describes the rationale and theoretical basis of a day program for clients with Alzheimer's disease. The program design is based on the principles of milieu therapy.

Topper, Joyce. "Adult Day Care in a Free-Standing Center." *O.A.H.A. Quarterly,* January 1985.

Describes briefly the activities within the program. Much of the discussion relates to the advantages and disadvantages of locating an adult day care program within a community recreational facility.

Index

Anxiety (*contd.*)
related to visuospatial deficit, 11.
See also Agitation; Fear
Apathy: appearance of, due to inertia, 14; due to lack of insight, 13–14
Aphasia: consequences of, 11; definition of, 10. *See also* Communication; Language; Language impairment
Appearance: attention to improving self-esteem, 127; awareness of, related to identity, 48; deterioration with dementing illness, 49
Apple tarts, recipe for, 57
Arguments, with clients, avoiding, 82
Armchair, use of, to facilitate seating, 102
Aromas, associated with activities, 55, 59, 60
Arrival: flexibility in client's arrival in program, 81; as part of program schedule, 40
Assembly line, arrangement of activities, 53
Assessment: of basic skills, 18; of behavior, 19; of client's abilities in relation to activity offered, 71. *See also* Evaluation
Assets, client's, identifying and using, 96
Attendance at program, limited to once weekly, 81
Attention: deficits in, 14; definition of, 14; maintaining client's, 72, 113
Autonomy: definition, 28; exercise of, through activity, 29

Babies, visiting program, 24
Basic needs, necessity of monitoring in dependent persons, 27
Basic skills, assessment of, 18
Beanbag toss, arranged as tournament, 48
Behavior: assessment of, 19; exam-

ple form for evaluating, 120; hostile and aggressive, 12; perplexing inconsistency of, in AD clients, 4
Birthdays, celebration of, in program, 66
Body awareness: contribution of grooming tasks to maintaining, 48; effects of deficit, 12, 109
Body language, as support for spoken language, 52, 113
Boredom, concern for clients' in program, 26, 114
"Busy work," questionable value of, 34

Car: facilitating entry and exit from, 102; use of staff vehicle to bring clients to program, 80, 93–94
Caregiver: emotional losses experienced by, 85; health evaluation of, 121; knowledge of disease process, 86; need to share feelings, 86; need for support, 83; visiting the program, 84; witness of client's stress, 83
Cerebral cortex, function of, 4–5
Cheese scones, recipe for, 56
Chili, recipe for, 54
Chores, housekeeping: as part of program, 52–53; importance of doing to client with AD, 29
Client's need to know about condition, 87
Clients least likely to benefit from group program, 81–82; alternatives for, 82
Coffee klatch: in daily schedule, 40; objective of, 108; as social time for clients, 51. *See also* Snack
Cognitive abilities, evaluation of, 123–24
Cognitive dysfunctions, list of most common, 109–10
Cognitive function, normal, 5–6
Color: client's perception of, as

required for activity, 37; as sensory stimulus, 37; use of, in program area, 31

Comfort, that clients provide to one another, 96

Commode, use of, to facilitate use of toilet, 102

Communication: with caregiver through journal, 84; consequences of deficient, 11; facilitating client's ability, 51–52; need for meaningful, 29; short sentences facilitating, 113

Communication sheet, with homemaker, sample, 118–19

Compensatory mechanisms: assessment of, 19; client's use of, to achieve higher level of function, 18

Competencies, client's, identified and transferred into home situation, 53, 126. *See also* Assets

Complaints, client's, to family about program, 94, 95

Conceptualization, client's difficulty with, 112–13

Confusion, paraphasia mistaken for, 10

Confusional state, superimposed upon dementia, 17

Continence: importance of body awareness in maintaining, 49–50; routine to maintain, 49. *See also* Incontinence

Contribution, clients' need to make, 52, 65

Control: definition, 28; grooming tasks as expression of, 49

Cookie cutters, use of small ones, 56

Cooking, as part of program, 53

Corridors, walking, 32

Crafts: basis for choosing, 58; examples of successful, 59–64; objectives of, 108; use at home of, 116

Croquet, modification to, 48

Cup of tea, making, used as evaluation, 90, 122

Daily notes, complement to initial evaluation, 20

Dance, as part of exercise program, 42

"Day Away": description of, 1; location in community of, 33; philosophy of, 2

Day programs, for Alzheimer victims, 1

Deficits, confronting client with own, 89

Demonstrations, use of, in program, 66

Denial, client's: of disease, 14; of problems 87–88

Dental hygiene, importance of, 49

Depression: associated with dementia, 18; mimicking dementia, 17

Design of program, definition, 30

Diagnosis, client's awareness of own, 91

Diagnostic procedures, ruling out other treatable conditions, 16

Difficult steps in activities, helping client with, 76

Embarrassment: client avoiding risk of, 75; resulting from client's poor judgement, 15; staff helping client avoid, 95

Emotions: providing outlet for, 24; rekindled by sensations, 25

Energy: clients' need for outlet of, 46; fluctuations in levels of, 38

Environment: assessment of client's home, 20; evaluation of, 16; physical, for program, 30–33

Errors, client's, coping with, 75–76

"Escape," dealing with clients attempting to leave, 81–82

Evaluation: done in home of client, 78; protocol example of, 120–26. *See also particular areas of evaluation*

Exercise period: aims of, 43; in daily schedule, 41; objectives of, 108

Exercise routine, 45–46

Exercises, helping client to perform, 44–45

Exits, demarcation of, in program area, 32–33

Expressive language: dysfunction, 10–11; evaluation of, 123

Facial expression. *See* Body language

Failure of activity: dealing with, 77; minimizing chances of, 38

Failure-proof activities, 61

Family Burden Index, use of, as part of assessment, 20

Family support, need for ongoing, 97

Family support groups, 97

Fear, client's: of change, 92; of failure, 70; of venturing out of the home, 80

Feeding fish, as one-step job, 53

Films, use of, in program, 66

Floors, in program area, 30

Flowers, pressed, use of, 62

Force, on clients: to attend program, 98; to participate in activity, 33

Forgetfulness vs. memory loss, 10

Functional evaluation, 18–19; form outlining, 122

Furniture: arrangement of, in program area, 31; clearly visible, 30

Furniture manufacturer, as source of materials, 64

Grooming: contribution to client's self-esteem, 48; in daily schedule, 41; as social time, 49

Gross motor activity: list of activities, 67; in program, 46–47

Guidance: importance of, 72; method of, 73–74; overview of, 110; providing meaningful, to client, 72. *See also* Help

Habitual abilities: definition of, 21; drawbacks to, 23; importance of, to client, 21; social skills as, 22; use of, in programing, 22, 74. *See also* Overlearned skills

Hand-over-hand direction, 73. *See also* Help

Hands-on direction, 110

Hazards in community, evaluation of, 121

Hazards in home: evaluation of, 120; identification of, potential, 20

Health history, sample of, 121

Health monitoring: importance of, 17; staff member's role, 51

Health risks, resulting from poor hygiene, 49

Help: how much to give, 73, 102; physical, giving to client, 73–74; verbal, giving to client, 73

Hierarchic Dementia Scale: caution in using, 89; as part of functional evaluation, 19

Home visit: established reason for, with client, 86; as important first contact, 78

Homemaker: client's acceptance of, in home, 96; introduction of, 93, 96–97; role of, with AD client, 112

Hostility, apparent in client, 12

Household chores: importance to clients, of doing, 52; list of activities, 67; use of, as home program activity, 115

Hygiene: attention to, as part of program, 48; family's difficulty in monitoring, 49

Identity: definition, 28; maintenance, through grooming activities, 48

Illness, causing sudden deterioration, 17

Impulsive behavior, embarrassment to client resulting from, 95

Inclusion: definition, 29; need for, addressed in sing-alongs, 51

Incontinence, possible reasons for, 49

Independence: assessment of, 18; form evaluating, 122; importance of, to client, 114; promoting client's sense of, 49, 60, 74

Independent living, assessment of, 19

Inertia: definition, 14; overcoming, 70–71; mistaken for apathy, 14

Initiation, client's deficit in, 109. *See also* Inertia

Injuries, minor, as alerts to potential dangers, 51

Instructions, use of, step-by-step, 74, 113

Intake assessment, family viewing, 90

Interpersonal relations, assessment of, 19

Introducing client to program, 78

Involvement, grading client's level of, 35

Ironing, as pleasant, familiar activity, 63

Journal: family's use of, 94; as part of ongoing evaluation, 20; as support to caregiver, 84

Judgment: consequences of, impaired, 15; deficit in, 110

Kitchen: designated area, 31; value of, in program area, 53

Labels, use of, in program area, 31

Language, evaluation of, 123

Language impairment: helping clients cope with, 52; kinds of, in AD, 10

Living conditions, sample form evaluating, 120–21

Location: choosing for activity, 70; of program in community, 33

Lunch time, objectives of, 108

Manicures, as part of program, 49

Manual direction. *See* help

Maslow, Abraham, hierarchy of needs, 27

Meal preparation: in day program, 53; list of activities, 67; used in activity program at home, 115

Memory: of emotional experiences, 8; memory related to senses, 7; parameters mediating, 7–9; problems in AD, 7; remote, use of, in programing, 25

Memory loss: embarrassment resulting from, 52; vs. forgetfulness, 10; frustration related to, 8; sparing client stress related to, 114; stress of, on caregiver, 10

Metaphors, failure to understand, 13

Mirror, one-way, use of, in program area, 84

Mobility: assessment of, 18; techniques facilitating, 100–102

Mobility deficits, related to spatial and postural insecurity, 99

Motor planning: deficit in, 109; need for, to function, 13

Movement: facilitated by use of rhythm, 24; normal, perceptual requirements of, 99; sense of, 24

Music, use of, 117

Needs: basic, 27; psychosocial, 28–29; security, 28

Negative feelings, client's: events contributing to, 95; as expressed to family, 84; about home visit, 78; retrospective, 91

Negative reaction, client's, persistent, to program, 81–82, 98

Negativism, perceived, reasons for, 70

Neurological examination, contribution to diagnosis, 16

Neuropsychological testing, importance of, 17

Seasonal events, in program schedule, 42

Seating, client in chair, method of, 101-2

Security, need for, and dementia as threat to, 28

Self-care: ability affected by disturbed body awareness, 12; assessment of, 18; home program activities, 115; list of activities, 67

Self-esteem: contribution of activity to client's, 37; definition, 29; grooming and hygiene, to build, 48; support of client's sense of, 112; threat to, of childish activities, 33

Sensory overload, avoiding, 24

Sensory stimulation: activities providing, 68; analyzing activity for, 37; importance of, 24; in program area, 31

Sequencing: accommodating client's difficulty, 70; deficit in, 13, 109

Shopping, as activity, 116

Signs, use of, in program area, 31

Sing-alongs, as social time for clients, 51

Snack: as part of program day, 40; cheese scones for, 56

Social activities: list of, 67; in program day, 51-52

Social history: importance of, in assessment, 20; sample, 121

Social isolation, 29, 85

Social skills: as habitual abilities, 22; maintained, to mask deficits, 85-86, 95; reinforced at snack time, 40

Space, use of, in program area, 31

Spaghetti sauce, recipe for, 55

Special events, in program, 66

Staff: to client ratio, 38-39; member, as consistent contact, 78

Stencils, use of, 64

Stereotypes, danger of adhering to, 15

Success: activities most likely to produce, 37-38; measurement of, 33

Suicide, client's threat of, 92

Task breakdown, importance of, 70, 74, 113

Time-out, clients' need for, 82

Van pick-up, as part of program day, 39

Verbal instructions, providing, 73, 110. *See also* Help

Visual prompts, use of, in communication, 52, 113

Visuospatial perception, definition and deficits in, 11-12

Voice quality, optimum when speaking, 113

Volunteer: education, outline of session, 107; in staff/client ratio, 38

Walker, facilitating client's use of, 100; use of, to stand, 101

Walking, as activity, 47, 116

Wind-down: as part of daily schedule, 42; as social time for clients, 51

Wood, as pleasant medium, 65

Woodwork, as program activity, 64-65

Work: as client's contribution to program, 65; list of activities, 68

Work area: selection of, 70; set up of, 54, 56, 57, 60

"Work bee" atmosphere, value of, 57, 60

Work table, covering for, 59